GP Tomorrow

Second Edition

Edited by

Jamie Harrison

and

Tim van Zwanenberg

Foreword by

Rebecca Viney

Joint-Chairman
GP Non-Principals Sub-Committee, GPC

Radcliffe Medical Press

Radcliffe Medical Press Ltd
18 Marcham Road
Abingdon
Oxon OX14 1AA
United Kingdom

www.radcliffe-oxford.com
The Radcliffe Medical Press electronic catalogue and online ordering facility.
Direct sales to anywhere in the world.

© 2002 Jamie Harrison and Tim van Zwanenberg

First edition 1998

British Library Cataloguing in Publication Data

A catalogue record for this book is available from the British Library.

ISBN 1 85775 560 X

Typeset by Acorn Bookwork, Salisbury, Wiltshire
Printed and bound by TJ International Ltd, Padstow, Cornwall

Contents

Foreword

I was honoured to be asked to write the foreword for this second edition of *GP Tomorrow*. The first edition was, without doubt, ahead of its time and this edition has been enriched, updated and has had new chapters added to it. The information within it provides a full understanding of the NHS changes and of the new forces driving the profession. This essential reading for new young general practitioners shows how we arrived here, and for established GPs it helps understand the demands made of new young GPs.

The book warns us that nobody should be complacent about the prospects for the future. Young doctors show many indications of becoming increasingly disillusioned. It is only their strong sense of vocation and commitment to patients that is preventing them from seeking other employment, which offers more reasonable working conditions. The provision of support and relevant education in the early years after training is essential, whether these young general practitioners are GP principals or non-principals.

To retain sufficient numbers of caring, competent and motivated doctors, these GPs must be encouraged to be life-long learners to avoid 'burn out'. To remain refreshed and keep developing they will need to be part of a 'learning society' as envisaged by the Dearing Report.

There has been a fall in numbers of doctors training for general practice since 1994. The loss is particularly marked in the inner cities and rural areas. Within these figures is concealed the fall in male applicants. Increasing numbers of GPs want to work part-time, take career breaks or earlier retirement. There is the apparent reluctance of new recruits to become principals. In London alone this year, the number of GP principals has fallen by 50. While many GPs may continue as self-employed, independent contractors, a significant and growing proportion will become salaried employees in the primary care trusts.

I believe this book is an essential tool for anyone involved in workforce planning, education and the new primary care organisations. It anticipates what will be required in the future, and the particular skills that GPs will need to learn continuously through their professional life, to adapt to change and sustain their enthusiasm and morale. Only when the individual doctor is healthy can he or she provide the quality practice that is required. The good doctor will maintain a balanced life despite continuing pressures from managers, patients and their own families. To do this they will make time for their own needs, 'for recreation, reflection and all that it means to be truly human'.

As well as being a workforce tool, this book manages to delight us – it reminds us about those things which matter and may not be measurable. It reflects on where we are and where we aspire to go and how we get there, and that it is an exciting time to be alive.

Rebecca Viney
Joint-Chairman
GP Non-Principals Sub-Committee
GPC
February 2002

Preface to second edition

Much has happened in the world of general practice since the original *GP Tomorrow* conference of October 1997. A new government has begun a modernisation programme. There is the *NHS Plan*. And being a salaried GP, taking a career break, or even leaving medicine altogether are no longer surprises.

The new enthusiasm for regulation and accountability, both professional and contractual, leaves many practitioners wary (and weary) of the latest directive from the centre. Yet there continues to be a steady stream of new GPs eager to develop personally and professionally, often as teachers and learners, utilising insights from other disciplines, not least the arts and humanities.

This second edition seeks to update many of the initiatives described in the first. In addition, the emergence of PMS posts and the developing role of GPs within the undergraduate medical curricula demand our attention. We remain grateful for the contributions of our colleagues, and for the continued patience, support and good humour of those with whom we work.

Jamie Harrison
Tim van Zwanenberg
February 2002

Preface to first edition

This book features contributions drawn mainly from amongst those who participated in a two-day conference held at the Royal County Hotel, Durham, in October 1997, entitled *GP Tomorrow*. The conference brought together general practitioners, including GP registrars, GP educationalists and GP academics, as well as health authority managers and representatives of the Royal College of General Practitioners and the British Medical Association.

The principal aim of the conference was to explore new initiatives in post-vocational training for general practice, particularly the schemes set up in Liverpool, London and Durham, responding to the question: 'How should we be training and nurturing the GPs of tomorrow?' Since the early 1990s it had become clear that young doctors leaving vocational training no longer rushed into joining traditional partnerships. They preferred to travel the world, do locums and take career breaks. The term 'generation X' has been used to describe this behaviour.

Yet a healthy scepticism about where general practice is heading, allied to an uncertainty about the future of work in its widest sense, is also being experienced by many existing general practitioners. Indeed, it is being recognised that, in a fast-changing society, the future role of doctors is no longer entirely predictable.

This book therefore addresses not just the needs of today's young practitioners, but also the question of how to equip all general practitioners for the challenges of the future. For tomorrow will still remain an uncertain country, but one in which general practitioners will retain a confident and honoured place.

We are grateful for the support and help of a wide variety of people in producing this book. In particular, we would like to thank all the contributors for their enthusiasm and hard work, and the many colleagues young and old who have stimulated our thinking. Angela McLaughlin has worked tirelessly and with great calm and good humour to produce the final typescript, and our considerable thanks are due to her.

Jamie Harrison
Tim van Zwanenberg
April 1998

How to use this book

We have deliberately set out to make reading this book a rewarding yet different experience for a wide audience, endeavouring to reflect the rapidly changing world of which the NHS is a part.

Content first. As general practice enjoys a central place in both the provision and commissioning of healthcare, its future is of interest to politicians, patients, health service managers and healthcare professionals, not least general practitioners. We have tried to include a range of these views, though inevitably our main focus has been the nurturing and development of general practitioners and their careers.

We have divided the book into three parts. The first (Chapters 1–6) sets the scene. Political and philosophical influences on general practice are traced and the importance of sound education and new technology emphasised. The second part (Chapters 7–12) describes a variety of practical initiatives which support general practitioners' professional development. The third part (Chapters 13–17) looks ahead, offering a critique of what doctors and patients might want for themselves and suggesting ways in which such a future might be achieved.

In a post-modern world you make your own rules ... which is what we suggest our readers do.

- You may wish to read the book from page 1 to the end.
- You may come with a particular interest, in which case we suggest you travel one of the three paths signposted overleaf.
- You may want to understand why younger doctors appear to have different expectations from older ones (Chapters 1 and 13).
- You may want to consider the significance of the changes in the NHS (Chapters 2 and 16).
- You may be interested only in practical examples (Chapters 7–12).

Choose your path

Patients	Doctors	NHS managers
Begin at Chapter 14 on what patients expect	Read Chapter 13 to see if you recognise doctors' views	Chapter 16 paints the future
↓	↓	↓
Try Chapter 6 to find out how GPs are trained	Go to Chapter 2 to explore the forces of change in the NHS	Chapters 7–12 describe practical initiatives
↓	↓	↓
Chapter 3 suggests you might have more of a say in the future	Chapter 1 puts it all in context with society at large	Chapter 15 suggests ways to help doctors
↓	↓	↓
Chapter 13 tells you how doctors feel	Chapters 7–12 describe practical initiatives	Chapters 13 and 14 give patients' and doctors' views
↓	↓	↓
Chapter 1 puts their feelings in context with society	Chapters 3, 15 and 16 paint the future	Chapters 3 and 6 give insight into GP training
↓	↓	↓
Read about practical approaches in Chapters 7–12	Remember patients are important. Read Chapter 14	Chapters 1 and 2 put it all in historical context

Contributors

Isobel Allen
Professor of Health and Social Policy, Policy Studies Institute

Lesley Delacourt
Independent Trainer and Management Adviser
Vocationally Trained Associates Co-ordinator

George Freeman
Professor of General Practice, Imperial College School of Medicine, London

Jon Fuller
Senior Lecturer, Department of General Practice and Primary Care, Imperial College School of Medicine, London

John Gillies
General Practitioner, Selkirk, Scottish Borders

Toby Gosden
Research Fellow, National Primary Care Research and Development Centre, Manchester

Jamie Harrison
General Practitioner, Durham and Associate Director of Postgraduate GP Education, University of Newcastle
Scheme Organiser, County Durham Health Authority GP Career Start

Sean Hilton
Head of General Practice and Primary Care, St George's Hospital Medical School, London

Brenda Leese
Reader in Primary Care Research, Centre for Research in Primary Care, University of Leeds

Jane Macnaughton
Director, Centre for Arts and Humanities in Health and Medicine, University of Durham

Virginia Morley
Senior Lecturer in Primary Care Development, Department of General Practice and Primary Care, King's College School of Medicine and Dentistry, London

Iain Mungall
General Practitioner, Bellingham, Northumberland

Roland Petchey
Director, Health Management Group, City University, London

Ian Purves
Head of Sowerby Centre for Health Informatics, University of Newcastle

Linda Redpath
Chief Officer, Community Health Council, Newcastle upon Tyne

Marianne Rigge
Director, College of Health

Richard Savage
General Practitioner and Course Organiser, Guy's and St Thomas' Vocational Training Scheme
Chair, South London Organisation of Vocational Training Schemes

Bonnie Sibbald
Professor, National Primary Care Research and Development Centre, Manchester

Frank Smith
Director of Postgraduate GP Education, Wessex

John Spencer
Professor of Medical Education in Primary Health Care, University of Newcastle

George Taylor
Director of Postgraduate GP Education, Yorkshire Deanery
Associate Dean, University of Leeds

Jacky Williams
Research Associate, Division of General Practice, University of Nottingham

Tim van Zwanenberg
Professor of Postgraduate General Practice and Director of Postgraduate GP Education, University of Newcastle

For our colleagues at
Cheveley Park Medical Centre, Belmont, County Durham,
and at
Collingwood Surgery, North Shields, Tyne and Wear

PART 1

Setting the scene

CHAPTER 1

Post-modern influences

Jamie Harrison

Presume not that I am the thing that I was.
Henry IV, part II

This chapter explores the changing relationships between doctors, medicine and society. In a post-modern world, traditional attitudes to life and work are questioned and new understandings suggested.

Changes in society

Contemporary Western society is at a crossroads. Conventional views about the meaning of vocation, career, marriage, work and sexuality face severe challenges. The nature of family life, the roles that men and women play and our understandings of why we are here are all up for discussion. In many ways, it is an exciting time to be alive. The confusion and uncertainty that such a fluid age brings, however, risk leaving some struggling to maintain their psychological equilibrium.

The generation that has dominated recent social developments and which finds itself now entering middle age is that born after the conflict of World War II. The marked rise in the birth rate, which followed the peace, led to the term the 'baby-boom' generation. Brought up in the 1950s, in closely supportive, nuclear families where wives did not work and divorce was rare, baby boomers became suffocated by restrictive customs and social practices.

One reaction to this cocooning, argues Karen Ritchie, was seen in the political and social upheavals of the 1960s, where a desire for freedom and change engulfed much of Western Europe and the USA.[1] The baby boomers went on to grasp the opportunities that post-war reconstruction offered to build their careers. Women in particular began to establish working patterns outside the home.

Generation X

The children of baby boomers are sometimes referred to as 'generation X', a generation born between 1961 and 1981.[2] They question many of their parents' assumptions and much of their value system:

> By 1990, the first of Generation X had finished their schooling and conceded that it would be necessary to work for a living and to play the game, as had every preceding generation. But they had already rejected both the rabid idealism of the 1960s and the excessive materialism of the 1980s. Xers vowed they would not sell out their friends, families or themselves in pursuit of a career, as Boomers had. Neither would they delude themselves that what they did for a living was more important than how they treated their neighbours or that the company they worked for demanded any special loyalty.[3]

The idea that there needed to be a proper balance between home, work and recreation was established. Work alone would no longer provide ultimate meaning in life (as had happened with baby boomers). Instead, it would complement relationships with friends and family, as well as fitting in to a larger philosophical framework. For many, this framework would have a post-modern feel to it.[4] This would be a generation concerning itself with major issues of conscience:

> Generation X ... see themselves as an alternative nation with alternative music representing alternative lifestyles. They have become content with living on less; desire more intimate relation-ships; are more embracing of diversity in race and gender; are more accommodating of social needs; and their individual identity is not based on what they accomplish, but rather on who they are.[5]

Post-modernity

Post-modern perspectives change the way we view the world. It looks and feels quite different. Dogmatic statements are questioned; image and perception are everything. Today is less certain and the future is what you make it. This shift in sensibility is captured by comparing the words used by modernists and post-modernists to describe their conceptions of how the world is designed (Box 1.1).

Box 1.1 Words to express a changing worldview

Modern	**Post-modern**
Purpose	Play
Design	Chance
Hierarchy	Anarchy
Closed	Open
Distance	Participation
Depth	Surface
Timeless	Passing
Order	Chaos
Control	Freedom
Certain	Fallible
Rigid	Flexible
Regulation	Deregulation

(Adapted from Harvey D (1995) *The Condition of Postmodernity*. Blackwell, Oxford)

Embracing a post-modern understanding of the world alters attitudes to work and a career. The future looks less clear-cut and many more fluid options open up. Risk-taking is more acceptable. Career changes and career breaks become necessary career components, rather than threats to future professional success. (This shift in thinking could have fundamental implications for future medical workforce planning.)

One major theme of post-modernity is its suspicion of master plans or generalisations.[6] This appears to undermine much of what medicine (as we know it) stands for − its career structures, hierarchies and traditions, as much as its dependence on rationality and the scientific method. Suspicion of the past leads us to reconsider the origins and development of modern medical practice and its practitioners.

The rise of modern medical practice

In many ways, science and, with it, scientific medicine has been the success story of the modern age. Yet how did this pre-eminence of scientific medicine arise? In the mid-19th century, before the development of the metropolitan general hospital, the majority of patients received their care in their homes on a private basis. Doctors had limited therapeutic tools, most of which were of unproven value. There was no medical monopoly. The medical profession was demoralised and lacked effective leadership, professional regulation, organisation and status.

What, then, happened to change the place of doctors in society? In Bryan Turner's view, the answer was the modern scientific revolution. For quite suddenly, 'surgery, treatment and hospitalisation became safe and effective'.[7] Advances in anaesthesia and antisepsis reflected a wider evolution of scientific medicine in Victorian Britain. The middle classes had money and status and wanted the best possible medical care for themselves and their families. Who can blame them?

> Between 1875 and 1920 ... the status of general primary care was greatly transformed and the social standing of the general practitioner was significantly enhanced. The growth in the demand for medical services was an effect of economic development, significant urbanisation and the evolution of an urban system of mass transport. The dominance and the autonomy of the medical profession was reinforced in this period by the growth of licensing laws which had the support of the state. A middle-class clientele developed with a specific demand for privatised scientific medicine, and furthermore the growth of an ideology of science greatly contributed to the receptivity of the population to technological medicine.[8]

By accepting a monocausal view of disease, grounded in the germ theory, both society in general and medicine in particular relocated their understanding of health and the origin of illness in a new wisdom. Victory over sepsis became the rallying cry. Health was defined as the absence of infection. Inevitable casualties flowed from this creed and not just among the microbes! Alternative ideas about the causes of illness and disease were discredited or forgotten. Social factors, such as poverty, the workplace, unemployment and poor housing, were left behind. The medical curriculum became dominated by a biomedical view and the specialist-led modern university medical school was soon to come of age.

Scientific medicine under threat

If the Golden Age of scientific medicine was between 1910 and 1970, with the rise of the district general hospital and the development of antibiotics, it is possible to see a crisis of confidence beginning to develop in the 1970s for both public and doctors alike. This partly reflected the very success of healthcare, as people lived longer and wanted ever more developed services.

Questions about the virtue and effectiveness of scientific medicine, however, seemed to be emerging even before any debate about rationing. As medicine struggled to fulfil its own promises, some patients and practitioners were beginning to wonder where the future for orthodox medicine might lie.

Indeed, new plagues had arisen as old ones found revived strength. It is not difficult to feel hemmed in by the supremacy of AIDS on the one hand and malaria, tuberculosis and cancer on the other. The secret – that medicine might be impotent in making any real difference in so many serious cases – was whispered. Its only protection was the over-optimism of some ('We'll find a cure/vaccine soon') or the collusive denial of others ('We're actually doing rather a good job'), supported by the macroeconomic interests of governments and pharmaceutical companies. The scientific success myth might live on, but some see gaps in the argument.

Questioning the relative strengths and weaknesses of the scientific approach should not be confused with the wholesale denial of the possibility of objectivity. Recent debate in the columns of the *British Medical Journal* emphasised that a post-modern suspicion of what is portrayed as scientific fact is exactly that – a suspicion, not an outright rejection.[9]

The rising tide of alternatives

A suspicion of beliefs, with its accompanying loss of certainty and questioning of authority, puts orthodoxy under the microscope. In medicine, both patients and doctors start to look beyond traditional models of medical care. Already, alternative, so-called complementary, therapies play an important part in healthcare. Their popularity appears to be on the increase as alternative therapists are able to give more time to their clients. A common complaint of patients is that their GPs offer too little time in the consultation. Offering something new, with a different set of rules governing the relationship between therapist and client, is attractive to both parties, not least to the GP complementary practitioner.

This blurring of roles has tantalising implications for general practice careers. Permission is granted for individual patients and practitioners to embrace alternatives without fear of ridicule. At one extreme, the general practitioner might leave scientific orthodoxy behind. At the other, whatever is scientifically unproven is rejected. What seems clear is that scientifically trained GPs are increasingly using alternative therapeutic options, either personally administered or by referral to others.

Such a world is not as unlikely as it first sounds. Back in 1962, Milton Friedman, Margaret Thatcher's guru, stated that: 'Licensure should be eliminated as a requirement for the practice of medicine.'[10] In such a world there would be no formal registration of medical practitioners. All providers would be welcome and the consumer left to decide. Such deregulation would fundamentally alter the hierarchical division between scientific and alternative medical approaches.

How the customer-patient decides the best and most appropriate treatment is of some significance. A pure market approach would presumably encourage experimenting with different options, with guidance being offered by advisers, regulators and consumer organisations. This would require a rethink of the traditional relationship between doctor and patient and the historically powerful position of the doctor would have to be scrutinised.

Power relationships

The doctor and patient

One particularly important critique that a post-modern perspective brings concerns the place of power and knowledge in professional relationships. The French historian-philosopher Michel Foucault sees power embodied in the everyday practice of medicine.[11] He questions how doctors and other health workers use their medical knowledge and privileged position to influence those they treat. Do they abuse their powerful position? Can they avoid the paternalism of old? Will they always act for the patient's good?

Confronted by a burgeoning choice of therapist and treatment, consumerist patients want a personal physician they can trust. No longer can the doctor claim authority by right. Respect must be won through an openly displayed desire to work for the patient's welfare. Something of this flavour of shared relationships is seen in the work of Hélène Cixous. She challenges doctor–patient relationships which are based on control and dependency and argues that such relationships fail to honour the gifts patients bring to the encounter – the vast amount of goodwill, trust and confidence they invest in their doctors. Here the doctor–patient relationship becomes one of open-endedness, trust and generosity.[12] This leads both doctor and patient to see the possibility for good in each consultation. This good has to be seen in the wider context of the GP role. General practitioners also perform the potentially compromising function of being gatekeepers to other services, which requires them both to ration services and act as patient advocate.

A good relationship allows an exploration of the complexity of medical options, interpreting for the patient what is possible, what is desirable and what the risks might be. In such transparent consultations, licensed doctors act with integrity, seeking to balance individual patient need, service capability and scientific evidence. Such doctors continue their privileged role by consensus and through agreement over what is true and trustworthy.

The clinical team

Doctors increasingly work in clinical teams, which bring their own difficulties for the individual patient. To whom does the patient look for guidance? What are the team dynamics? Do some members of the team abuse their powerful position for their own ends? This theme of the potential abuse of power has been taken up by Dr John Parboosingh of the Royal College of Physicians and Surgeons of Canada. He speaks of doctors in a changing world, such that:

> Doctors must also be taught to manage change and accept that power is a privilege not a right; that their role is not necessarily to head teams but to be influential members of them.[13]

The power of a doctor in the team can suffocate dialogue and impose a prejudiced view. By examining their pre-suppositions about what they know and believe and why, doctors can engage with colleagues and patients in a truthful dialogue. This is not the same as the doctor merely offering all the available treatment options without being willing to participate in the discussion as a serious engaged professional. That is the negation of responsibility.

Rethinking the way we live

Doctors, as much as patients, are reassessing what is important *for them* in a changing world. This refocusing involves both home and workplace and beyond. The traditional stereotype of the general practitioner – white, male and career dominated, expected to fulfil certain expectations of self and patients alike – is under review. The large detached house used to mark affluence and success. The doctor's wife would not work professionally, other than in answering the telephone or perhaps by performing occasional reception duties. Children attended boarding schools outside the practice area, a large estate car being used to transport their belongings to and fro.[14]

Ecological conservation and a simpler lifestyle now appear more necessary and attractive. A value system with greater emphasis on sustainability and a sharing of power and authority prevails. This approach to life manifests itself in the concept of being a *world citizen*, rather than a *global consumer* (Box 1.2).

Box 1.2 Values for the world

Global consumer	**World citizen**
Me	We
More	Enough
Materialism	Holism
Quantity	Quality
Greed	Need
Short term	Long term
Rights	Responsibilities

(*Source*: *Who Needs It?* SustainAbility (1995))

Here, the fundamental value is that of holism, rather than materialism. To have enough is enough and the drive to ever greater acquisition and status is not well developed. Indeed, it is consciously rejected. Such a post-materialist worldview fits the idea of a mosaic society, in which networking and stake-holding predominate. It is the world of the corner shop and the bicycle, rather than the superstore and the two-car household (Box 1.3).

Box 1.3 Downshifting – risk and mosaic societies

Risk	**Mosaic**
Consumerism	Post-materialism
Shareholder value	Stakeholder value
Volatile income	Citizen's income
Two-car household	Two-bike household
Superstore	Corner shop
Personal computing	Network computing
Go for it	Get a life
Working harder	Working smarter
Economic growth	Sustainable development
Self-reliance	Mutuality
Workaholism	Search for balance

(*Source*: The Henley Centre for Forecasting)

Implications for GP tomorrow

The shift away from a work-dominated and consumerist approach to life appears healthy, as long as the basic financial demands for living are met. For GPs there are options, e.g. they can share a two-doctor list between three partners; time for education and relaxation is scheduled in the week; family commitments are slotted into the programme; housing remains modest; holidays are not over-expensive; and schooling is local and state-funded.

Other GPs will seek a different lifestyle, with the freedom to purchase quality housing, a large garden and access to private education. They will work extremely hard to maintain their standard of living. The question is not about which way of life is better, but rather about the extent to which such variations in how we live affect and shape future work and career patterns.

The old dominance of a particular medical career may be passing and multiple choices and opportunities will present. This is the world of the GP tomorrow.

Conclusion

As a new millennium begins, it is no longer possible to be certain of finding the world of medicine at peace with itself. Equally, society at large is beginning to question the role of the medical profession and its ability to perform the miracles once expected.

Governments now find deregulation attractive, whether for corporations or state monopolies. Society craves high standards and answers to the questions it poses on health and disease. Communication has never been easier and we all demand our rights – the best is only (just) good enough.

The GPs of tomorrow will not be able to relax back into the old ways of doing things. Nostalgia may be attractive, but the world has moved on, as has the new generation of doctors. They are no longer willing to accept sloppy standards, poor working conditions, minimal continuing medical education and poor professional support. They are willing to say that things must be different and demand change.

Some have labelled them the 'slackers' generation. They are accused of being work-shy, looking for low-paid jobs without responsibility (McJobs). This view has been refuted with vigour.[15] Generation Xers are prepared to put in the necessary hours (and effort), but they need a say in the purpose of the work and demand proper training, career options and flexibility. They will not follow blindly or just do things because 'this is how we have always done it'.

Summary

- Baby boomers are over-committed to work.
- Generation Xers seek to balance career, home and recreation.
- Post-modern thinking questions whether science has all the answers.
- Alternative therapies risk undermining traditional medical models.
- Doctors have a powerful position in society.
- Patients bring goodwill and trust to the consultation.
- New trends in society affect doctors as they do others.
- Tomorrow's GPs will demand training, support, career options and flexibility.

References

1   Ritchie K (1995) *Marketing to Generation X*. Lexington Books, New York.

2   Explored in Coupland D (1992) *Generation X: tales for an accelerated culture*. Abacus, London; see also Harrison J and Innes R (1997) *Medical Vocation and Generation X*. Grove Books, Cambridge.

3   Ritchie *op cit.* pp. 104–5.

4   The definition of the term 'post-modern' is fluid; one definition might be 'an all-pervasive mood and not a rational structure; a shift in sensibility'. See Huyssen A (1986) *After the Great Divide: modernism, mass culture, postmodernism*. Indiana University Press, p. 181. For a general introduction, Appignanesi R and Garratt C (1995) *Postmodernism for Beginners*. Icon Books, Cambridge.

5   Gerali S (1995) Paradigms in contemporary church which reflect generational values. In: P Ward (ed) *The Church and Youth Ministry*. Lynx, Oxford.

6   Described by the French philosopher Jean-François Lyotard as a suspicion of 'grand narratives' – those overarching systems of belief which explain how things are.

7   Turner BS (1990) The interdisciplinary curriculum: from social medicine to postmodernism. *Sociology of Health & Illness*. **12**: 1–23.

8   ibid. pp. 7–8.

9   Hodgkin P (1996) Medicine, postmodernism and the end of certainty. *BMJ*. **313**: 1568–9; see also Letters, Harrison J (1997) Doctors have a duty to remain true patient advocates. *BMJ*. **314**: 1044–5.

10   Friedman M (1962) *Capitalism and Freedom*. University of Chicago Press, Chicago.

11   Lupton D (1997) Foucault and the medicalisation critique. In: A Peterson and R Bunton (eds) *Foucault, Health and Medicine*. Routledge, London.

12   Fox NJ (1993) *Postmodernism, Sociology and Health*. Open University Press, Buckingham, p. 68.

13   Richards T (1997) Disillusioned doctors. *BMJ*. **314**: 1705–6.

14 This atmosphere is well captured by Blake Morrison (1993) in *And When Did You Last See Your Father?* Granta Books, London.

15 Tulgan B (1996) *Managing Generation X: how to bring out the best in young talent.* Capstone, Oxford.

CHAPTER 2

Strategic shifts

Tim van Zwanenberg

What's past is prologue.
The Tempest

This chapter traces the changes in general practice since the inception of the NHS in 1948. It suggests that there have been a number of 'strategic shifts', including a shift of power and influence towards general practice. Further change in the way primary care is organised is inevitable.

In recent years general practitioners have found themselves placed in an increasingly pivotal position in the NHS. Yet general practice has not always enjoyed or exercised significant power and general practitioners' enhanced influence on the NHS has been matched by other changes, which are just as strategically significant – for example, the rise of consumerism and the potential created by advancing technology.

Box 2.1 The ages of NHS general practice

The Dark Ages	1948–66 • Single-handed and on call at all times. • Home as surgery and wife as receptionist. • Income from capitation only.
The Renaissance	1966–86 • Group practices and primary healthcare teams. • Better premises. • Academic departments.

The Reformation	1986–90
	• New GP contract.
The Market	1990–97
	• Strategic shift to primary care.
	• GP commissioning.
	• Community-based services.
Modernisation	1997–
	• Collaboration in new primary care organisations.
	• Collective clinical governance.
	• Individual accountability through appraisal and revalidation.

The Dark Ages

The self-esteem of those who have pursued a career in general practice has fluctuated widely since the inception of the NHS in 1948 (Box 2.1). In the early years, general practitioners typically worked on their own, used their home as a surgery and relied on their wives (for they were almost exclusively men) to receive callers and to answer the phone. They were on call at all times and were paid by capitation, that is, the number of patients on their list.

In 1950, in his 30-page seminal report in *The Lancet*, Collings concluded that:

> My observations have led me to write what is indeed a condemnation of general practice in its present form; but they have also led me to recognize the importance of general practice and the dangers of continuing to pretend that it is something which it is not. Instead of continuing a policy of compensating for its deficiencies, we should admit them honestly and try to correct them at source.[1]

Collings also claimed that general practice was a unique social phenomenon and that general practitioners enjoyed more prestige and yielded more power than any other citizen 'unless it be the judge on his bench'. He surmised that the powers of even senior managers were petty in comparison to doctors' influence on the physical, psychological and economic destiny of other people. The general practitioner's power, however, was confined to individual patients and was therefore of little importance to the organisation of the health service.

The 'importance of general practice' was not to be recognised for some years and general practice remained in the doldrums for the 1950s and early 1960s. The perception that GPs were failed hospital doctors pervaded the medical establishment, and morale among GPs was extremely low. Many UK graduates emigrated to North America and general practice in most urban areas was only sustained by an influx of doctors from overseas, mainly from the Indian subcontinent.[2]

The Renaissance

In 1966 both the profession and the government recognised the pressing need for change. As a result of the *Charter for the Family Doctor Service, a* new contract for GPs heralded major developments of the service.[3] A new three-part payment system of basic practice allowances, capitation fees and item-for-service payments was supplemented by group practice allowances and incentives for doctors to work in under-doctored areas. Partial reimbursement of the salary costs of practice clerical and nursing staff was instituted and funds were made available for the building or upgrading of premises.

These measures increasingly fostered the formation of group practices, the employment of ancillary staff such as receptionists and practice nurses, the development of premises and an expansion in the range of services offered to patients, for example surgery-based nursing care. As long ago as 1920, the Dawson Report on community healthcare had recommended that local health authorities provide, equip and maintain health centres where groups of doctors and other healthcare staff could work in collaboration.[4] Yet by 1966 only 28 purpose-built group practice premises had been developed, housing only about 200 general practitioners in total.[5]

It now became more normal for district nurses and health visitors to be attached to practices. Vocational training for GPs was expanded, becoming mandatory in 1982, and academic departments of general practice were established in most medical schools. The Royal College of General Practitioners (RCGP), which had been established in 1952, increased its membership (by examination) and steadily enhanced its reputation as the guardian of standards in practice.

If general practice has ever had a Golden Age, it was probably between 1975 and 1986. In this period the self-confidence of the discipline grew and general practice was the first-choice career for many of the brightest graduates. Those who wished to develop their practices largely had the freedom to do so.

The Reformation

The pace of development of general practice over the two decades following the Charter was, however, far from uniform. A series of reports, particularly from the RCGP, beginning with *What Sort of Doctor?*,[6] identified considerable variations in the quality of care provided by different practices. This did not go unnoticed by politicians, who were quite able to draw their own conclusions from seeing single-handed lock-up shop surgeries in some parts of the inner cities.

Although the government did not pursue the introduction of the good practice allowance, first mooted in the 1986 Green Paper on primary care,[7] it did not abandon its aims of making services more responsive to the needs of the patient and of raising the standards of care. And these have been persistent themes of government policy ever since, irrespective of political party. By 1990, mainstream GP influence on government policy appeared to reach its nadir, with the imposition of a new and highly contentious (and contended) contract for GPs.[8] The 1990 contract made GPs more accountable for what they did, and even then the government was accused of trampling on their professional autonomy and of imposing clinical direction.[9]

Among general practitioners it was said that, whereas the 1966 contract helped the good to get better, the 1990 contract was framed to control the bad. In the event, some gains, for example improved uptake of immunisation and cervical smear screening and the introduction of medical audit, were offset by many losses. Health promotion clinics were ridiculed for their bureaucracy and ineffectiveness, yet many practices increased their income by instituting them. There was scant evidence to support either annual health checks for the elderly or examinations for those who had not seen a general practitioner in three years.[10] The information provided in the mandatory practice annual reports was rarely used for interpractice comparisons, nor did it feed into individual practice development. Arguably the 1990 contract was the inevitable result of the combined effect of a disunited profession and a frustrated government.

The Market

In parallel with the introduction of a new contract, general practitioners also had to contend with a radical reform of the NHS. The White Paper *Working for Patients*[11] concentrated on achieving better use of available NHS funds, through the creation of a competitive internal market with the separation of purchaser and provider. Health costs were expected to fall and the quality of service to rise. For markets to achieve this, however, supply must exceed demand. This was not, is not and never will be the case with the NHS, where demand far outstrips supply.

Although general practitioners had been badly bruised by the 1990 contract, their influence and power would grow considerably as a result of GP fundholding and its later variants – community fundholding, total purchasing and locality commissioning.[12] GP fundholding, in particular, created a potential means of transferring both clinical activity and resources from the secondary to the primary care sector. It also appeared to release considerable creative energy among general practitioners for the benefit of their patients.

GP fundholding was not without its disadvantages. There were lasting concerns about equity, with allegations of preferential funding, and the transaction costs were high, with a cumbersome information system. Whatever conclusion may ultimately be drawn about GP fundholding, it did signal a significant shift in the balance of power within the NHS – a shift that would be sustained even when fundholding was later abolished.

One side effect of GP fundholding would prove something of a barrier to the future recruitment of general practitioners. GP fundholders were able to use fundholding savings to extend and upgrade their premises, so adding to the value of the capital assets of the partners. In future, new partners would need to borrow a much larger sum in order to buy their share of the partnership premises. Disputes about the valuation of such premises and the issue of negative equity would make entering a partnership increasingly complicated.

Paradoxically, in spite of general practitioners' increased role in providing and commissioning care, morale appeared to reach a low point in the mid-1990s. Was this because they really wanted to be clinicians and small business people and not public health physicians or managers?

Whatever the truth behind this paradox, in 1996 the Conservative government, now with a very small majority and not apparently in the mood for radical or unpopular change, engaged the profession in a consultation – the so-called 'Listening Process'. The upshot was new enabling legislation, the Primary Care Act, based on the White Paper *Primary Care: the future. Choice and opportunity.*[13] This allowed the government to suspend NHS regulations for pilot projects approved by the Secretary of State. These projects explored different ways of organising primary care, including the provision of salaried general practitioner posts. The incoming Labour government was to use this legislation for its own purposes in developing Personal Medical Services – as opposed to General Medical Services regulated by the national GP contract – as a way of creating different contractual arrangements for NHS general practitioners.

Modernisation

Between the inception of the NHS in 1948 and May 1997 then, there had been incremental development in general practice and a strategic shift towards primary care. But the incoming Labour government had a very large parliamentary majority and a mandate to 'modernise' the public services. Furthermore, quality in the NHS in general and the regulation of doctors in particular were to become major political priorities, as a series of cases of doctors' misdemeanours unfolded, creating lurid headlines in the popular press.

Two of these cases have had the most profound effects – Bristol and Shipman. In June 1998, after the longest-ever hearing before the General Medical Council, two senior doctors at the Bristol Royal Infirmary, James Wisheart and John Roylance, were struck off, and restrictions placed on a third doctor's practice. The then Secretary of State for Health famously criticised the General Medical Council for failing to strike off all three accused doctors.[14] In January 2000 Hyde general practitioner Harold Shipman was convicted of murdering 15 of his patients. It was suspected that he had murdered many more, and Professor Richard Baker, in his report for the Department of Health on Shipman's practice, concluded he had certified 297 'excess' deaths.[15]

Against this background of crisis and change there was a raft of new policy initiatives in the years following the Labour election victory of 1997, from both the government and the profession. Furthermore, with increasing political devolution, real differences in NHS structures and processes began to emerge among the four countries in the United Kingdom. For the sake of simplicity the English versions are cited here, while recognising that our colleagues in the other three countries are finding the language of the English NHS increasingly alien. The following policy documents are of relevance to the future general practitioners.

A Review of Continuing Professional Development in General Practice[16]

This report defined continuing professional development as:

> 'a process of lifelong learning for all individuals and teams which enables professionals to expand and fulfil their potential and which also meets patients' needs and delivers the health and health care priorities of the NHS'.

Its principal recommendation was that general practices should compile Practice Professional Development Plans (PPDPs), and that these should initially run in parallel with and ultimately replace the existing Postgraduate Education Allowance (PGEA) system, whereby general practitioners were paid for attending accredited courses. The PPDP would be based on the service development plans of the practice, local and national NHS objectives, and identified educational needs. Individual development plans for all members of the practice team would be incorporated, and would reflect both practice priorities and individual career aspirations. The plan would use practice-based and other novel forms of learning and give an indication of measures of success. Further guidance for primary care was promised but never materialised.

The New NHS: modern, dependable[17]

In this White Paper the government outlined a range of policy initiatives, which would have an effect on the role, responsibilities, accountability and regulation of general practitioners, including:

- the abolition of GP fundholding (which had been voluntary and only ever achieved about 50% coverage of general practitioners)
- the formation of primary care groups, of which all general practitioners had to be members, which were to:
  - contribute to health authorities' Health Improvement Programmes
  - promote the health of the local population
  - commission health services
  - monitor performance
  - develop primary care
  - better integrate primary and community health services
- the creation of a new 24-hour telephone advice service, *NHS Direct*, staffed by nurses
- the development of a national performance framework for the NHS
- the introduction of clinical governance (backed by a new statutory duty for quality in NHS organisations)
- the development of a programme of new evidence-based National Service Frameworks setting out the patterns and levels of service which should be provided for patients with certain conditions
- the establishment of a new National Institute for Clinical Excellence to promote clinical and cost-effectiveness by producing clinical guidelines and audits for dissemination throughout the NHS
- the establishment of a new Commission for Health Improvement to

support and oversee the quality of clinical governance and clinical services
- the development of work with the professions to strengthen the existing systems of professional self-regulation
- the introduction of a new national survey of patient and user experience.

A First Class Service: quality in the new NHS[18]

In this Green Paper the government elaborated its policy framework, through which standards for the NHS would be set, delivered and monitored (Table 2.1). This placed professional self-regulation alongside clinical governance and lifelong learning as the methods of local delivery.

Table 2.1 Setting, delivering, monitoring standards

	Quality mechanism
Clear standards of service	• National Institute for Clinical Excellence • National Service Frameworks
Dependable local delivery	• Professional self-regulation • Clinical governance • Lifelong learning
Monitored standards	• Commission for Health Improvement • National Performance Framework • National Patient and User Survey

Supporting Doctors, Protecting Patients[19]

This was a consultation paper from the Chief Medical Officer on 'preventing, recognising and dealing with poor clinical performance of doctors in the NHS in England'. In it he suggested that it had not been clear how the quality assurance activities of the medical bodies (General Medical Council and Medical Royal Colleges) under the auspices of professional self-regulation related to the similar responsibilities discharged by the NHS. He also pointed out that general practitioners, as independent contractors, could not be suspended by health authorities, even in serious circumstances, and that the only way a general practitioner could be removed from NHS practice was via the NHS Tribunal (unless they had been struck off or suspended from the Medical Register by the General Medical Council). This was the case no matter what the nature of the problem – indecent assault, fraud, mental health problem or dangerous practice.

The document included the following proposals.

- Participation in clinical audit as part of clinical governance should be compulsory for all general practitioners.
- Appraisal should be made comprehensive and compulsory for all doctors working in the NHS.
- Present disciplinary procedures should be replaced, and new procedures should extend to all doctors including general practitioners.
- A new independent Performance Assessment and Support Service should be established (ultimately the National Clinical Assessment Authority).
- Any referral to it should result in a range of outcomes: a period of re-education and training; referral to the General Medical Council; referral for medical treatment; referral back to the employer with a report that the problem was serious and intractable. In the latter case the doctor would be dismissed.
- Health authorities should be given a new power to suspend general practitioners.

A Health Service for All the Talents: developing the NHS workforce[20]

This consultation document stemmed from 'long-standing concerns about the way in which the NHS educates, trains and uses its staff'. It proposed that in the future the emphasis needed to be on:

- team working across professional and organisational boundaries
- flexible working to make best use of the range of skills and knowledge
- streamlined workforce planning and development which 'stems from the needs of patients not of professionals'
- maximising the contribution of all staff to patient care, 'doing away with barriers which say only doctors or nurses can provide particular types of care'
- modernising education and training

- developing new, more flexible, careers for staff of 'all professions and none'
- expanding the workforce to meet future needs.

The NHS Plan. A plan for investment. A plan for reform[21]

This was the plan of NHS reform with a timetable and targets to accompany the massive injection of extra funding, which had been announced by the Chancellor of the Exchequer in March 2000. Among its many proposals the following would have an impact on general practitioners.

- A major expansion in Personal Medical Services would be encouraged, with the development of a national core Personal Medical Services contract, and work with the profession to amend the national GP contract (for General Medical Services) in a similar way. The revised national contract 'should reflect the emphasis on quality and improved outcomes inherent in the Personal Medical Services approach'.
- All doctors working in primary care, whether principals, non-principals or locums, would be required to be on the list of a health authority and be subject to clinical governance arrangements. These would include annual appraisal and mandatory participation in clinical audit.
- A National Clinical Assessment Authority would be established as a Special Health Authority to provide a rapid and objective expert assessment of an individual doctor's performance, recommending to the health authority educational or other approaches.
- The NHS Tribunal would be abolished, and the power to suspend or remove general practitioners from a health authority's list devolved to health authorities.
- By 2004, patients would be able to see a primary care professional within 24 hours and a general practitioner within 48 hours.
- Up to 1000 specialist general practitioners would be developed to take referrals from fellow general practitioners for conditions in specialties such as ophthalmology, orthopaedics and dermatology.
- The further development of primary care trusts into care trusts to provide even closer integration of community-based health and social care services.
- The Commission for Health Improvement, with the support of the Audit Commission, would inspect every NHS organisation every four years.
- NHS occupational health services would be extended to general practitioners and their staff.

- By 2004, a single phone call to *NHS Direct* would be the 'one-stop gateway' to out-of-hours healthcare, passing calls on where necessary to general practitioners.

The plan also promised increased numbers of general practitioners, 2000 more by 2004, and increased numbers of doctors training to be general practitioners, 450 (later increased to 550) more by 2004.

Revalidating Doctors: ensuring standards, securing the future[22]

This consultation document finally set forth the General Medical Council's proposals for revalidation, and identified a three-stage process.

1 A folder of information describing what the doctor does and how well the doctor does it. This would be regularly reviewed – annual appraisal would fulfil this in many sectors.
2 Periodic revalidation – a recommendation by a group of medical and lay people that the doctor remains fit to practise, or that the doctor's registration should be reviewed by the General Medical Council.
3 Action by the General Medical Council – in the majority of cases, revalidation of the doctor's register entry. In a minority, detailed investigation under the council's 'fitness to practise' procedures, which can lead to restrictions on practice, suspension or erasure.

The General Medical Council confirmed that doctors' performance was to be assessed against the principles laid out in *Good Medical Practice*. These principles were grouped under seven headings – good clinical care, maintaining good medical practice, relationship with patients, working with colleagues, teaching and training, probity, and health. Appraisal was seen as the central process and its link with revalidation was described. It was proposed that revalidation should take place every five years.

Impact of policy changes

The years following the Labour election victory thus saw a series of policy developments affecting or potentially affecting the contractual and/or professional regulation of general practitioners, including, for example, compulsory participation in annual appraisal, compulsory participation in primary care groups, changes in the arrangements for continuing professional development, possible suspension by a health authority, possible referral to the National Clinical Assessment Authority, compulsory participation in clinical audit, routine inspection by the Commission for Health Improvement, and finally, obligatory quinquennial revalidation. These developments were accompanied by major structural changes, not least in the planned constitution of the General Medical Council and in the establishment of four new national bodies (in England) – the Commission for Health Improvement, the National Institute for Clinical Excellence, the National Clinical Assessment Authority and the National Patient Safety Agency. The consequence of all these changes is that all general practitioners in the future, both principals and non-principals, can anticipate a markedly different professional life.

Strategic shifts in the NHS

The growing influence of general practitioners and the extension of community-based services are but two of a number of 'strategic shifts', which have underpinned the NHS at the turn of the millennium (Box 2.2) and which are visible mainly in retrospect. These shifts represent movement and change in strategic or overall direction.

Box 2.2 Strategic themes in the NHS at the turn of the millennium

Value for money	• efficiency • equity • more for less
Quality	• clinical effectiveness • clinical governance
Engaging with patients	• information for patients • patients' involvement • patients' rights and responsibilities
More influence for general practitioners	• GP fundholding • locality commissioning • primary care trust commissioning
More community-based services	• extension of primary care • *NHS Direct* • GP specialists • hospital at home • hospital outreach

---

Value for money

The change of government in 1997 made no difference to the drive for value for money (efficiency) which had been the basis of the Conservatives' NHS reforms. In fact, in common with healthcare systems across the world, there has been a consistent move to 'get more for less'. Equity has also now been reintroduced as a guiding principle (the NHS had, after all, been created with the objective of reducing inequity). An emphasis on financial equity would at least help challenge variations in clinical practice, and lead to clinical equity. [23] It remains to be seen whether this can be achieved, but it leads on to the issue of quality.

Quality

Quality has been a recurring theme, albeit under a number of different guises – medical audit, clinical audit, health gain, clinical outcomes, (unacceptable) variations in practice, evidence-based medicine, clinical effectiveness, clinical governance and clinical excellence! The notion of benefit has come to pervade much of the rhetoric of the NHS. The NHS reforms had brought with them the widespread introduction of medical audit (later called clinical audit to encompass the multidisciplinary approach to healthcare). Medical audit induced considerable anxiety amongst general practitioners, who feared external inspection and imposition of standards. However, most medical audit advisory groups (MAAGs), which were established in each district, were able to dispel these fears and promote practice-based and problem-oriented audit. A more recent perceived threat, evidence-based medicine, is now in the process of being absorbed into general practice, with general practitioners recognising that the evidence from randomised controlled trials (RCTs), in particular, needs to be incorporated judiciously into consultations with patients.[24]

But still more is wanted by the government as part of the development of clinical governance in the NHS. The implications of this responsibility being shouldered locally are slowly being determined. General practitioners, as participants in the new primary care groups and trusts, are having to develop new skills both in monitoring and assuring the quality of care provided by their colleagues.

Engaging with patients

Patients want more than just information; they need involvement too.[25] And patients have had something to say, though their involvement in the

NHS and its decision making has often suffered from pious exhortation and tokenism.

Improved engagement with patients represents another strategic shift in emphasis for the NHS, with the idea of a partnership with patients gaining ground. There have been a number of elements to this: providing patients with better information; hearing patients' views on plans and services through questionnaire surveys, focus groups, citizens' juries and community health councils; involving patients in quality assurance; and establishing a number of explicit rights for patients through the Patient's Charter.

Patients are more ready to complain and to express their views on how their care should be organised. The rapid growth in sources of information, from self-help groups, books, telephone helplines and the media, means that patients are better informed not only of their rights but also about their illness and its treatment. It is not uncommon for patients attending their general practitioners to produce a printout of information about their illness from the Internet.

Even better access to information and much greater participation in quality assurance are forecast as being what patients will expect in the future (Chapter 14).

Driving forces

These shifts in the strategic direction of the NHS have not come about by accident. There has been a range of forces driving change across society and all societal institutions. The NHS is not immune to these forces, which might be summarised as:

- cost
- technology
- consumerism
- political theory.

No healthcare system in the world is stable and it is predicted that the pace of change is unlikely to relent. Indeed, some believe that our health system will probably see more changes in the next two decades than in the past two. Most large sectors of developed economies – transport, manufacturing and retail – have been transformed since 1980. It is argued that healthcare has not, but that it will be.[26]

The rising cost of healthcare interventions and the changing demography of the population, with increasing numbers of very elderly people, mean that, whatever the success of any preventive programmes, the cost to the NHS will rise. The shift to primary care may have been driven by policy founded on the premise that services in the community are intrinsically cheaper to provide. The evidence for this belief is difficult to find, though obvious in its simplest form. The cost of one day of hospital inpatient care is in general much more expensive than the cost of care provided at home. The real equation, of course, is not so simple.

Technology and the development of sophisticated medical procedures have led to the 'compression of morbidity' (patients recover more quickly from illness and surgical procedures) and greater reliance on ambulatory care (patients walk in and walk out the same day). In the 1970s, for example, patients stayed in hospital for a week or so for a hernia repair. Now more than 90% of such operations are carried out as day-case procedures. It is hard to envisage the future changes that will result from advances in genetics, telemedicine, robotics, information technology and pharmaceuticals.

Patients as consumers are better informed, more litigious and, some would say, health obsessed. They are part of a consumerist society, which is in general more affluent (but with an alienated underclass concentrated in poor urban areas). The traditional single-income two-parent nuclear family as the norm in society is at an end. Consumerism is pressing on all providers of goods and services, including those like the NHS in the public sector.

The dominant political theory of the last two decades, competition, is being superseded by a more collective and collaborative approach.[27] It remains to be seen whether this will suit general practitioners and whether they will be able to act more corporately through primary care trusts. Failure to do so may see their power and influence wane as managers reassert their decision making on behalf of the local population.

Future organisation of primary care

For many general practitioners, their ideal is a well-organised training group practice in spacious premises with a full primary healthcare team providing and commissioning a wide range of high-quality services for their patients. Yet there are practices that provide poor clinical care and a limited range of services while the general practitioners cultivate a policy of high list size and high personal income. Some practices still waste resources through high rates of referral, poor prescribing and inappropriate use of investigations.[28] Increasingly the NHS will begin to tackle these unacceptable variations in practice, through primary care trusts' clinical governance activities, and through quality-based contracts.

The remains of our past healthcare system, and not least its remarkable achievements, exert great inertia on any plans to redesign the NHS for the future – an NHS which can respond to the needs and wants of patients, practitioners and government alike. What perhaps most bedevils attempts to re-engineer the health service is the overwhelming legacy of its current structures. The most obvious of these are the large city and district general hospitals, the product of healthcare policies of a past age. Yet these hospitals are the capital estate of the NHS and institutionalise much of the care provided within them. Equally, the provision of primary care is governed by long-standing assumptions about the general practitioners' monopoly on provision, exercised through patient registration and the list system.

The combination of the Primary Care Act (with its consequent Personal Medical Services examining new ways of providing primary care) and the formation of new primary care organisations commissioning 75% of hospital care mean that more change, and possibly very radical change, is on the way. And although the strategic emphasis on primary care remains, the challenges are considerable.

Future changes in the organisation of general practice and primary care will need to address:

- increasing consumer demand for services, information and involvement
- increasing public, professional and government pressure for greater transparency, accountability and demonstration of high standards of care
- continuing upward pressure on cost.

The practice partnership as the basic unit of delivery may soon have reached the limit of its capacity, particularly in urban areas. For it no longer makes sense, nor is it efficient, for the NHS to sustain a large number of small outlets each with their own administrative systems and each handling a very large turnover of public funds. Local primary care organisations (trusts) serving, say, 100 000 people could take their place, absorbing local practices as they develop. Such organisations may use the techniques of managed care more efficiently; ensure a more consistent quality of service; be better placed to assess and reduce risks; and provide greater career flexibility for staff of all kinds. The organisation would oversee staff induction, in-service training, continuing professional development and governance of the clinical care provided.

Conclusion

The strategic shift to primary care still has some way to go. It is being driven by forces that operate across society as a whole. The partnership model of general practice may no longer suffice in all areas and new kinds of primary care organisation are emerging.

Among the many challenges that the predicted organisational upheavals may bring, none will be greater than maintaining general practice as a discrete discipline – a discipline which defines itself in terms of relationships, especially the relationship between patient and doctor.[29]

Summary

- There has been a shift of power and influence towards primary care.
- Government policy is not the only driving force.
- Technology and patient preferences play a part.
- The only certainty is more change, particularly in the way primary care is organised.
- The practice as the basic unit may have reached the limit of its capacity.

References

1   Collings JS (1950) General practice in England today: a reconnaissance. *Lancet.* 1: 555–85.

2   Wilkin D, Halham L, Leavey R and Metcalfe D (1987) *Anatomy of Urban General Practice.* Tavistock Publications, London.

3   British Medical Association (1965) *Charter for the Family Doctor Service.* BMA, London.

4   Consultative Council on Medical and Allied Services (1920) *Future Provision of Medical and Allied Services. Interim Report (Chairman: Lord Dawson).* HMSO, London.

5   Drury VWM (1977) Premises and organisation. In: J Fry (ed) *Trends in General Practice.* RCGP, London.

6   Royal College of General Practitioners (1985) *What Sort of Doctor?* RCGP, London.

7   Secretaries of State for Social Services, Wales, Northern Ireland and Scotland (1986) *Primary Health Care: an agenda for discussion.* Cmnd 9771. HMSO, London.

8   Department of Health and the Welsh Office (1989) *General Practice in the National Health Service. A new contract.* Department of Health and the Welsh Office, London.

9   Lewis J (1997) The changing meaning of the GP contract. *BMJ.* **314**: 895–8.

10 Scott T and Maynard A (1991) *Will the New GP Contract Lead to Cost-effective Medical Practice?* York Centre for Health Economics, University of York.

11 Secretaries of State for Health, Wales, Northern Ireland and Scotland (1989) *Working for Patients.* Cmnd 555. HMSO, London.

12 Glennerster H, Cohen A and Bovell V (1996) *Alternatives to Fundholding.* London School of Economics, London.

13 Secretary of State for Health (1996) *Primary Care: the future. Choice and opportunity.* HMSO, London.

14 Warden J (1998) Dobson criticises GMC. *BMJ.* **316**: 1925.

15 Department of Health (2001) www.doh.gov.uk/hshipmanpractice

16 Department of Health (1998) *A Review of Continuing Professional Development in General Practice.* Department of Health, London

17 Department of Health (1997) *The New NHS: modern, dependable.* The Stationery Office, London.

18 Department of Health (1998) *A First Class Service: quality in the new NHS.* The Stationery Office, London.

19 Department of Health (1999) *Supporting Doctors, Protecting Patients.* Department of Health, London.

20 Department of Health (2000) *A Health Service for All the Talents: developing the NHS workforce.* Department of Health, London.

21 Secretary of State for Health (2000) *The NHS Plan: a plan for investment, a plan for reform.* The Stationery Office, London.

22 General Medical Council (2000) *Revalidating Doctors: ensuring standards, securing the future.* GMC, London.

23 Bevan G (1998) Taking equity seriously: a dilemma for government from allocating resources to primary care groups. *BMJ.* **316**: 39–43.

24 Sackett DL, Rosenberg WMC, Gray JAM, Haynes RB and Richardson WS (1996) Evidence based medicine: what it is and what it isn't. *BMJ.* **312**: 71–2.

25 Richards T (1998) Partnership with patients. *BMJ.* **316**: 85–6.

26 Smith R (1997) The future of healthcare systems. *BMJ.* **314**: 1495–6.

27 Innes R (2001) Modernisation and New Labour. In: J Harrison, R Innes and T van Zwanenberg (eds) *The New GP: changing roles and the modern NHS.* Radcliffe Medical Press, Oxford.

28 Pringle M (1997) An opportunity to improve primary care. *BMJ.* **314**: 595–7.

29 McWhinney IR (1996) The importance of being different. *British Journal of General Practice.* **46**: 433–6.

CHAPTER 3

The changing consultation

Ian Purves

The future belongs to the unreasonable man who looks forward, not back, who thinks the unthinkable and who is certain only of uncertainty.
GB Shaw

This chapter explores new ideas about the consultation and the incorporation of evidence-based medicine. It suggests the computer will be an inevitable third party in consultations in the future.

Pastoral care or evidence-based medicine?

The post-modernist world of general practice is a mixture of the medieval world of pastoralism, renaissance activities revolving around evidence-based medicine and the new world of the information age. This diversity lacks a cohesive exploration of the issues. Individual clinicians are unable to develop a personal philosophy in which they can bring these issues together and develop a modern consultation style.

The declining influence of the church in the Western world has led members of society seeking 'guidance' for living to approach new sources of advice. The Balint movement of the 1970s brought general practice into pastoral care and attempted to align it with scientific method. Understanding and addressing the psychosocial issues of illness are much to do with the art of general practice. Some, such as Peter Sowerby, have lamented the 'loss' of the developing scientific method, while recognising the role of Balintism.[1] The holistic approach to general practice has moved on. Patient-centred clinical method has refined and progressed the art of general practice.[2-5] But can it be sustained without balancing the art with the science?

Clinical epidemiology, as the science of the art of medicine, has been rebadged as evidence-based medicine. The continuing process of defining an evidence-based approach has been complicated by the semantics of the word 'evidence'. Many in general practice, with its domain of 'life, the universe and everything', have resisted the redefinition. In the evidence-based movement there is debate around how to incorporate patient preferences into the decision-making process.[6] A further aspect of the science of the art is an understanding of the role of narratology in development of the consultation.[7,8] Narratology is the term used to denote the 'branch of literary study devoted to the analysis of narratives, and more specifically of forms of narration and varieties of narrator', where narrative is telling of some true or fictitious event or connected sequence of events recounted by a narrator to a narratee (although there may be more than one of each). A narrative consists of a set of events (the story) recounted in a process of narration (or discourse), in which the events are selected and arranged in a particular order (the plot).

These separate debates, on the art and the science of the art of medicine, proceed without any unifying understanding of the role of each in general practice. Meanwhile, the whole nature of medicine is being turned on its head with the information age and the informed participative society.[9]

Consultation in general practice

To move the general practice consultation forward, we need to understand the role of general practice and the role of the consultation. We need to grasp how to become more evidence-based in the consultation and why the information age is developing 'unorthodoxy' in our patients. We need to consider a new clinical method in the consultation, while looking into the near future to see how professional boundaries need to be blurred.[10]

The nature of general practice can be described as identifying problems (whether they are presented or asymptomatic), classifying the problem and understanding the impact of the illness on the individual. Thence the problem is resolved or ameliorated to the patient's satisfaction, within the bounds of medical capabilities and society resource limitations, while helping the individual to cope and manage their illness.

The consultation is a scene with the lead actors in the health drama – the patient/carer representing a health/illness need and the clinician representing general practice. Within the consultation:

[T]he task of the patient is to convey his health beliefs to the clinician; and of the clinician to enable this to happen. The task of the clinician ... is to convey her (professionally informed) health beliefs to the patient; and of the patient, to entertain these. The intention is to assist the patient to make as informed a choice as possible about diagnosis and treatment, about benefit and risk and to take full part in a therapeutic alliance.[11]

Incorporating the evidence

As early as 1876, Huxley, speaking on medical education in the House of Commons, predicted the expansion of medical knowledge beyond that which is absorbable by individuals. For general medicine, it has now been quantified. The clinician needs to read 17 articles a day every day of the year and this number can be predicted to be much larger in general practice.[12] Until recently, expert reviews[13] or phone calls to friends in secondary care[14] have been the source for general practitioners resolving uncertainty about their professional health beliefs. Of course, the expert is known to be unable to express his or her expertise in an unbiased way.[15] Nor can the expert explain why something is so, as well as what should be done. This has been called the 'paradox of expertise'.[16] Human beings often rationalise their behaviour without recognising that their explanations as to why they are behaving in a certain way are frequently wrong.[17] Here the role of evidence-based medicine comes to the fore, with its transparency of process of systematic reviews and its validity of why a recommendation is so derived from meta-analysis.[18]

There has been some criticism of evidence-based medicine in general practice.[13,19] It is true that randomised controlled trials have selected populations, often drawn from secondary care, that do not match the real world. There is a shortage of good evidence about the conditions commonly seen in general practice. Evidence focuses on classified abstractions (diagnoses) rather than individuals. And if practised as proposed on a case-by-case basis (Box 3.1), which could take at least two hours per case,[20] the caseload of the average general practitioner will need to be significantly reduced.

Box 3.1 Four steps in evidence-based medicine (adapted from Rosenberg[20])

- Classify the patient's problem then formulate a clear clinical question.

- Search the literature for relevant clinical articles.
- Evaluate (critically appraise) the evidence for its validity and usefulness.
- Implement useful findings in clinical practice.

However, evidence-based medicine is misunderstood:

> Evidence-based medicine is a conscientious, explicit, and judicious use of current best evidence in making decisions about care of individual patients. The practice of evidence-based medicine means integrating individual clinical expertise with the best available external clinical evidence from systematic research.[21]

Clinical expertise and evidence

In future, doctors in consultation need to be clearer about the role of clinical expertise and the role of 'best available external clinical evidence'. Given the time constraints in general practice, access to evidence needs to be easy and pre-digested to individuals' (clinician and patient) characteristics. Evidence-based guidelines,[22,23] especially the computerised form,[10,24–28] seem to be a key part of the solution. Developments in computing and health informatics should enable narrative description of the 'clinical question' and synthesis of relevant research. However, at present research publications are written in the 'wrong way' and guidelines remain the critical route to evidence. This difference between clinician and researcher is a 'cognitive mismatch'.[29] The mismatch occurs because researchers work in an analytical mindset with well-structured tasks, whereas clinicians work in an intuitive mindset with unstructured tasks.[30] We need computerised guidance that matches the pattern recognition process that clinicians, as experts, use in the consultation.[30] Of course, guidelines do not always cover the breadth or depth of knowledge that clinicians and patients may require to resolve uncertainty. Hypermedia* knowledge bases need to be linked to clinical guidance to help clinicians explore a depth of knowledge that would initially overload them in order to help resolve any uncertainty they may have with the

---

***Hypermedia**: the World Wide Web on the Internet is a well-known form of hypermedia with text, 'hotlinks' to other documents, pictures, sound and video.

presented guidance.[27] Hypermedia may also be a useful tool to broaden the initial clinical thought process.

Although there is a sense of inevitability and logic in evidence-based medicine, there are still nagging doubts. What is the 'evidence' of clinical expertise? This is difficult to validate, yet by understanding the cognitive model of expertise,[29] the role of stories in understanding the whole patient,[31] decision making[32] and education,[33,34] my current hypothesis is that health narratology[7] will become part of the science of the art of medicine. In such a way, we can start to use 'evidence' that respects expertise and the developing, more formal definition of evidence.

Patients and evidence

The patient clearly has more time to focus on his or her illness than the doctor. In the information age the individual could undertake (or have some patient group researcher undertake) an evidence-based search, leaving the poor clinician with a manifest gulf in his or her knowledge. So the patients could become more empowered – but do they want to be? Many general practitioners believe that patients want them, as informed clinicians, to make the decisions. It is worth exploring general practitioners' paternalistic beliefs and some beliefs that patients have about the consultation. Cromarty[35] found that:

> ... patients thought most about the problems that led them to the surgery, but they also considered their situation, particularly the available time and the behaviour of the doctor. To a much lesser extent, they considered matters that the doctor introduced. Underlying all these thoughts was continuous reflection and interpretation – a search for meaning.

The issue of time is not one of satisfaction but one of maintaining a personal relationship with an adviser.[35–38] However, this relationship is not left unchallenged.[35] Patients do interpret and compare the view of the doctor with other opinions that have been offered. It has already been shown that the GP as a source of health information is in decline, especially among younger age groups.[39] Doctors seem unaware that patients discriminate about the value of medical opinions. Patients present a selective discourse towards the 'orthodox' view of medicine even when considering 'unorthodox' actions (Table 3.1).[11,40]

Table 3.1 Orthodoxy and unorthodoxy of patients

Orthodox	Unorthodox
Doctor sanctioning of patients' behaviour	Self-legitimisation
Obedience to doctor	
Doctors as experts	
Scientific legitimisation	Anti-drug attitudes
	Medicine as unnatural and harmful
Doctors under-prescribe	Doctors over-prescribe

The unorthodox view is increasingly being proffered by the media, especially by investigative journalism.[40] If soap operas pick up the thread of these unorthodox views they might be expressed by even more patients.[41] Furthermore, it would be reasonable to assume that the inherent developing tribalism that comes with the information age might spawn disease-specific 'tribes' and further enhance this trend to unorthodoxy.[42] Experimental models like the Wisconsin AIDS Patient Virtual Community using the Comprehensive Health Enhancement Support System (CHESS)[43,44] can already be seen to be developing groups of ill individuals with a kindred spirit which are partly self-supporting. It is clear to me and others that paternalism has little role in the modern consultation.[11,40,45] The only exception to this rule is where expectations of the older generations make it impossible to share responsibility with the individual patient.

If patients are to benefit from correct decisions about diagnosis and management, they need to be educated about their problem(s) and the benefits and risks of the therapy. In this way they will be able to share management decisions.[11,46] Once a shared decision has been made, the patient needs: further detailed education about the therapy; to be motivated; and to have potential barriers assessed to enable concordance between the health beliefs of the clinician and patient.[11,47] Self-care is critical if there is to be a better therapeutic alliance between the clinician and patient. Compliance with medication currently ranges around 50–75%![11]

Time and teamwork

It seems likely that future consultations will be longer than the current 5–10 minutes. Do we need to increase the number of general practitioners? There is no straightforward answer to this. There is no simulation model available able to predict the effects of any of the following realities.

- Informed patients will undertake self-care with assistance from physical and virtual (e.g. CHESS) support networks. Medicine needs to find its (legitimate and important) role. Consultations will decline.
- The age of the population is increasing and there will be increased chronic ill health. Consultations will increase.
- Patient education and chronic disease monitoring is not a natural role for general practitioners. More consultations will be shared across the team.
- Personal care is a major determinant of patient satisfaction.[48] Core primary care teams need to be small (one general practitioner, one nurse and one secretary?).
- Constant flux in the organisation of the healthcare system will reduce the need for and ability of general practitioners to manage small health enterprises. There will be more clinical time available. Those interested in management will be remunerated and recognised accordingly.

What will general practice look like? This is difficult to predict, but the requirements appear straightforward – nested groups of small teams, perhaps not dissimilar from what we have in the UK already. Personal lists of around 2000 patients may be covered by a doctor, a nurse and a secretary, or group practices with a population of around 10 000 will have a wider clinical team (physiotherapist, counsellor, pharmacist, health visitor, midwife, etc.). Administration may be reduced by communities of group practices working together to manage all or almost all healthcare resources of a population of around 100 000–250 000. It is important that any model supports the lowest common denominator in the healthcare system – the consultation. This raises the issue of teamworking, the definition of roles of different clinicians, their relevant clinical activity and record taking, and other 'groupware' issues (see below).

Interdisciplinary working with trust, tolerance and a willingness to share responsibility is critical to teamwork.[49] To enable effective training, we do need to be aware of the core skills and knowledge required for each role. The key to being a general practitioner is knowing individuals and their families before they become ill. Once they become ill the general practitioner needs to think of the patient as an individual rather than a generalised abstraction (diagnosis), but still be able to categorise the abstraction at a level which ties the psychosocial in with the physical (problem).[50] Once the problem has been identified, the GP needs to educate the patient and make a shared decision about what (if any) intervention should be undertaken. The feature that makes a general practitioner unique (even in the medical domain) is the ability to sort the unsorted – differentiate the undifferentiated problem within the domain of life, the universe and everything. The nurse in general practice is neither 'handmaiden' nor 'technical functionary'[51] but an independent practitioner skilled at listening, explaining and understanding, with a key role to play in prevention and chronic disease management through guidelines.[50,52] The primary care nurse also has the same holistic nature as the general practitioner. Both types of clinician need personal but professional health belief models. Neither can be replaced by each other, lay individuals or computers (ever).

Teamwork and the computer

It has been easy to propose teamworking and even to claim its existence, but is there a primary care team? Some research suggests it is rarer than claimed.[53] Working as teams or groups is well studied. Small personal groups are most effective[54] and computer software has been shown to promote effective group working. This software is called groupware – a 'computer-based system that supports groups of people engaged in a common task (or goal) and that provides an interface to a shared environment'.[55] A primary care team should have a common philosophy and share common tasks and goals. Those tasks and goals need to be communicated and co-ordinated.[56] In the dispersed environment of the community and with a health system adding barriers, for example the primary–secondary care interface, groupware can engender a shared environment. Some aspects of groupware important to the future consultation can be seen in Box 3.2.[57] The computer is becoming part of the healthcare team.[10]

Box 3.2 General practice groupware (the three Cs)

Communication

- patient health records for the whole team
- email
- clinical electronic data interchange (EDI)
- telemedicine.

Collaboration

- team guidelines and other knowledge bases
- team-based clinical audit
- computer-based educational resources.

Co-ordination

- monitoring the status of actions/tasks
- scheduling resources and tasks.

Patient-centred consulting

Most of this chapter has been about the context of the consultation rather than the activity within a consultation. The consultation is a deeply personal activity which is dependent on the:

> ... physicians' personalities and their perceptions of themselves and their tasks ... If we are on the brink of a transformation of clinical method we are also on the brink of a change in the way physicians think and feel.[3]

What sorts of thoughts and feelings are important? When discussing diseases, doctors are generally reminded of individuals. Conversely, the medical school clinical method focuses on diagnosis which distances us from experience.[50] Caring and healing are not about categories but about individuals' stories. We still need these abstractions, however, for making causal inferences and applying modern interventions. We should not split the 'body' from the 'mind'. We need to understand the mind–body as a person's story. This leads us to:

> The essence of the patient-centred method ... the doctor attends to feelings, emotions and moods, as well as categorizing the patient's illness ... The key skill is attentive listening.[50]

Attentive listening is but part of the whole picture. To attend to the patient's feelings and emotions we need to be self-aware. One of the biggest challenges is self-reflection.[50]

The patient-centred method[2–5] remains a key to healing as the 'restoration of wholeness' (Box 3.3).[3]

Box 3.3 The six interactive components of the patient-centred process

- Exploring both the disease and illness experience.
- Understanding the whole person.
- Finding common ground regarding management.
- Incorporating prevention and health promotion.
- Enhancing the patient–doctor relationship.
- Being realistic.

The patient-centred approach is not the whole of the consultation. *Cum scientia caritas* (scientific skill with loving kindness) is the motto of the Royal College of General Practitioners. Although scientific skill is implicit in the patient-centred approach, it is often not expressed clearly. Science and experience must live together so we can see the patient as a whole. Perhaps it is the legacy of Balint and the attempt at scientific 'legitimisation' of the psychosocial that has stopped this clear expression.[1] But we can hold both the science and the art together through narrative. For this to happen, the clinician and patient need to be part of the same story – experiencing the illness and sharing the scientific facts.

Triadic consultations

As highlighted earlier, the information requirements for shared decision making are greater than the cognitive capacity of clinicians. Some form of information support is required. Computer guidance for clinicians and hypermedia-shared information resources will be needed. To enable teamworking, groupware is needed to promote a shared understanding of tasks/goals and to create a shared environment. This means that a computer needs to become the third member in the triadic relationship of the consultation.[10] In the UK, the computer is already used by 81% of general practitioners in some consultations (33% in all consultations). Seven per cent of general practitioners are paperless (another 16% are effectively paperless but hang onto the Lloyd George envelopes). Yet only 29% use the computer for guidance and 12% for email.[58] Having used them for some time, 78% of general practitioners believe computers could enhance their ability to deliver best practice. It is to be noted that 66% feel they need training to enable them to consult with the computer.[58]

Given the important human issues raised about the nature of the consultation, should we allow this 'natural' progression towards the triadic consultation or should we call a halt now? The debate rehearsed in this chapter provides two possible (and diametrically opposed) answers.

- No – the consultation dynamics are too precious and will be disrupted.
- Yes – the science of the art is too demanding without the computer and the patient will become more 'informed'.

Accepting that training about minimal effective use of the computer is possible, that there appears to be no other effective way of handling the information explosion and that, arguably, computers will become ubiquitous and part of the human story, it is up to health informaticians to make them as transparent as is both legitimate and possible.

From this, a new set of interactive components for the future consultation can be proposed (Box 3.4). These components are laid out in semisequential fashion but consultations are rarely so simple. To help envisage the tasks to be performed within the consultation, I have listed them sequentially for a simple consultation in Box 3.5.

Box 3.4 The interactive components of the future consultation

- Exploring the story to categorise the problem and understand the illness experience and patient health beliefs.
- Balancing the evidence of experience and up-to-date research findings using clinical information systems.
- Explaining professionally informed health beliefs to the patient.
- Enabling the patient to make an informed management decision being aware of the benefits and risks of potential therapy through possible shared computer interaction.
- Engendering self-care through assessment of motivation and barriers, having realistic goals plus reinforcement of professional health beliefs over time.
- Incorporating prevention and health promotion.
- Enhancing the healing relationship between the individual and clinician.
- Making adequate electronic notes of the story to enable teamwork.

Box 3.5 A task model for the clinician within a 'simple' consultation

- Reading the story – viewing the information on computer (pre-consultation), listening, observing, examining and directing conversation.
- Understanding the story.
- Utilising the clinical information system with the patient.
- Discussing the options (perhaps referring to other team members for further discussion).
- Setting the therapeutic actions in motion through the clinical information system.
- Writing the story (post-consultation).

The future can only involve continual change. We cannot forecast what the information age will bring nor how quickly. Furthermore, changes in the organisation of the NHS could have a significant impact.

The biggest issue facing general practice is professional attitude. We will need to become more self-reflective, perhaps through a better education in philosophy, art and classics, but certainly with better support networks and reflective time. Education is lifelong and we need to learn skills from evidence-based practice, narratology and health informatics to support our continual learning. Computer systems need to develop to support and not hinder the consultation. We need training in bringing the computer into the story. Finally, we need to develop and foster small personal teams for the individual patient through tolerance, trust and shared responsibility rather than hierarchical 'delegation'.

I think the future is bright – the future of healthcare lies in the primary care consultation.

Summary

- General practice consultations involve both the art and the science of the art of medicine.
- Evidence and expertise need to be balanced and incorporated in the consultation.
- Understanding the patient and their story is critical.
- Information technology can support both evidence-based decision making by patients and doctors, and teamworking.
- The computer is an inevitable third party to the consultation.

References

1 Sowerby P (1977) The doctor, his patient, and his illness: a reappraisal. *Journal of the Royal College of General Practitioners.* **27**: 583–9.

2 Pendleton D, Schofield T, Tate P and Havelock P (1984) *The Consultation: an approach to learning and teaching.* Oxford University Press, Oxford.

3 McWhinney IR (1986) Are we on the brink of a major transformation of clinical method? *Canadian Medical Association Journal.* **135**(8): 873–8.

4 Levenstein JH, McCracken EC, McWhinney IR, Stewart MA and Brown JB (1986) The patient-centred clinical method. 1. A model for the doctor–patient interaction in family medicine. *Family Practice.* **3**(1): 24–30.

5 Stewart MA, Brown J, Weston WW *et al.* (1995) *Patient-centred Medicine.* Sage Publications, London.

6 McPherson K (1994) The best and the enemy of the good: randomised controlled trials, uncertainty, and assessing the role of patient choice in medical decision making. *Journal of Epidemiology and Community Health.* **48**: 6–15.

7 Kay S and Purves IN (1996) Medical records and other stories: a narratological framework. *Methods of Information in Medicine.* **35**: 72–88.

8 Kay S and Purves IN (1998) Putting the narrative medical record in its place. In: T Greenhalgh and B Hurwitz (eds) *Narrative Based Medicine: dialogue and discourse in clinical practice.* BMJ Publications, London.

9 Smith R (1997) The future of healthcare systems. *BMJ.* **314**: 1495–6.

10 Purves IN (1996) Facing future challenges in general practice: a clinical method with computer support. *Family Practice*. **13**: 536–43.

11 Marinker M (ed) (1997) *From Compliance to Concordance: achieving shared goals in medicine taking*. Royal Pharmaceutical Society of Great Britain, London.

12 Davidoff F, Haynes B, Sackett D and Smith R (1995) Evidence based medicine. *BMJ*. **310**: 1085–6.

13 Taylor R (1996) Experts and evidence. *British Journal of General Practice*. **45**: 268–70.

14 Smith R (1996) What clinical information do doctors need? *BMJ*. **313**: 1062–8.

15 Sackett D (1983) Proposals for health sciences. I – Compulsory retirement for experts. *Journal of Chronic Disease*. **36**: 545.

16 Johnson PE (1983) What kind of system should an expert be? *Journal of Medicine and Philosophy*. **7**: 77–97.

17 Musen MA (1993) An overview of knowledge acquisition. In: JM David, JP Krivine and R Simmons (eds) *Second Generation Expert Systems*. Springer-Verlag, Berlin.

18 Egger M and Smith GD (1997) Meta-analysis: potentials and promises. *BMJ*. **315**: 1371–4.

19 Risdale L (1996) Evidence-based learning for general practice. *British Journal of General Practice*. **46**: 503–4.

20 Rosenberg W and Donald A (1995) Evidence based medicine: an approach to clinical problem solving. *BMJ*. **310**: 1122–6.

21 Sackett D, Rosenberg W, Muir Gray JA, Haynes RB and Richardson WS (1996) Evidence based medicine: what it is and what it isn't. *BMJ*. **312**: 71–2.

22 Eccles M, Clapp Z, Grimshaw J *et al*. (1996) Developing valid guidelines: methodological and procedural issues from the North of England Evidence Based Guideline Development Project. *Quality in Health Care*. **5**: 44–50.

23 Grimshaw G, Eccles M and Russell IT (1995) Developing clinically valid practice guidelines. *J Evaluation Clinical Practice*. **1**: 37–48.

24 Grimshaw JM and Russell IT (1993) Effect of clinical guidelines on medical practice: a systematic review of rigorous evaluations. *Lancet*. **342**: 1317–22.

25 Johnston ME, Langton KB and Haynes RB (1994) The effects of computer based clinical decision support systems on clinician performance and patient outcomes. A critical appraisal of research. *Annals of Internal Medicine*. **120**: 135–42.

26 Sullivan F and Mitchell E (1995) Has general practitioner computing made a difference to patient care? A systematic review of published reports. *BMJ*. **311**: 848–52.

27 Purves IN (1995) Computerised guidelines in primary health care: reflections and implications. In: C Gordon and JP Christensen (eds) *Health Telematics for Clinical Guidelines and Protocols*. IOS Press, Amsterdam.

28 Purves IN (1998) PRODIGY: implementing clinical guidance using computers (editorial). *British Journal of General Practice*. **48**: 1552–3.

29 Dowie J (1994) *The Research-Practice Gap and The Role of Decision Analysis In Closing It*. European Society for Medical Decision Making, Lille.

30 Schmidt HG, Norman GR and Boshuizen HPA (1990) A cognitive perspective on medical expertise: theory and implications. *Academic Medicine.* **65**(10): 611–21.

31 Daniel SL (1987) Literature and medicine: in quest of method. *Literature and Medicine.* **6**: 1–12.

32 Mattingly C (1991) The narrative nature of clinical reasoning. *American Journal of Occupational Therapy.* **45**(11): 998–1005.

33 Calman KC (1997) Literature in the education of the doctor. *Lancet* **350**: 1622–4.

34 Hunter KM (1991) *Doctors' Stories: the narrative structure of medical knowledge.* Princeton University Press, Princeton, NJ.

35 Cromarty I (1996) What do patients think about during their consultations? A qualitative study. *British Journal of General Practice.* **46**: 525–8.

36 Branthwaite A (1996) The image of the patient in their relationship with general practitioners. *British Journal of General Practice.* **46**: 504–5.

37 Baker R and Streatfield J (1995) What type of general practice do patients prefer? Exploration of practice charateristics influencing patient satisfaction. *British Journal of General Practice.* **45**: 654–9.

38 Baker R (1996) Characteristics of practices, general practitioners and patients related to levels of patients' satisfaction with consultations. *British Journal of General Practice.* **46**: 601–5.

39 Griffin JP and Griffin JR (1996) Informing the patient. *Journal of the Royal College of Physicians of London.* **30**(2): 107–11.

40 Britten N (1996) Lay views of drugs and medicines: orthodox and unorthodox accounts. In: SJ Williams and M Calnan (eds) *Modern Medicine: lay perspectives and experiences.* UCL Press, London.

41 Smith BH and Taylor R (1996) Medicine – a healing or dying art? *British Journal of General Practice.* **46**: 249–51.

42 McLuhan M and Powers BR (1989) *The Global Village: the transformations in world life and media in the 21st century.* Oxford University Press, Oxford.

43 Gustafson DH, Bosworth K, Hawkins RP, Boberg EW and Bricker E (1992) CHESS: a computer-based system for providing information, referrals, decision support and social support to people facing medical and other health-related crises. *Proceedings Annual Symposium Computer Application in Medical Care.* 161–5.

44 Gustafson DH, Hawkins RP, Boberg EW and Bricker E (1994) The use and impact of a computer-based support system for people living with AIDS and HIV infection. *Proceedings Annual Symposium Computer Application in Medical Care.* 604–8.

45 McKinstry B (1992) Paternalism and the doctor–patient relationship in general practice. *British Journal of General Practice.* **42**: 340–2.

46 Horne R (1997) Representations of medication and treatment: advances in theory and measurement. In: KJ Petrie and JA Weinman (eds) *Perceptions of Health and Illness.* Harwood Academic Publishers, Amsterdam.

47 Green LW (1987) How physicians can improve patients' participation and maintenance in self-care. *Western Journal of Medicine.* **147**(3): 346–9.

48 Baker R (1997) Will the future GP remain a personal doctor? *British Journal of General Practice*. **47**: 831–4.

49 Nolan M (1995) Towards an ethos of interdisciplinary practice. *BMJ*. **311**: 305–7.

50 McWhinney IR (1996) The importance of being different. *British Journal of General Practice*. **46**: 433–6.

51 Denner S (1995) Extending professional practice: benefits and pitfalls. *Nursing Times*. **91**(14): 27–9.

52 Koperski M, Rogers S and Drennan V (1997) Nurse practitioners in general practice – an inevitable progression? *British Journal of General Practice*. **47**: 696–8.

53 Bond J, Cartlidge AM, Gregson BA *et al.* (1987) Interprofessional collaboration in primary health care. *JRCGP*. **37**: 158–61.

54 Øvretveit J (1993) *Coordinating Community Care: multidisciplinary teams and care management*. Open University Press, Buckingham.

55 Ellis CA, Gibbs SJ and Rein GL (1991) Groupware: some issues and experiences. *Communications of the ACM*. **34**(1): 39–58.

56 Freeman G (1984) Continuity of care in general practice: a review and critique. *Family Practice*. **1**(4): 245–52.

57 Purves IN (1995) Decision support at the primary/secondary care interface. In: P Pritchard (ed) *Decision Support in Primary and Secondary Care*. NHS Executive R&D, London.

58 Purves IN (1998) *General Practice Computerisation National Survey 1996*. NHS Executive, Leeds.

CHAPTER 4

What can undergraduate education offer general practice?

John Spencer

This chapter explores how medical students are taught in the community and reflects on how the future might be different.

Introduction

Trainers and GP registrars alike have long recognised that vocational training is essentially a remedial process. Whether straight out of pre-registration house jobs, or some time later, the hapless registrar must undergo a major reorientation to the new environment and a considerable amount of 'unlearning'. Those entering general practice after a hospital career may require intensive rehabilitation. This is not a new phenomenon. Historically medical school curricula were required to produce doctors capable of independent practice, literally on the day after graduation, yet those entering general practice, on the whole, have always found themselves ill equipped to do the job.

A little bit of history

In fact there were repeated calls from the 1950s onwards for more teaching to take place in general practice. A report by the Undergraduate Education Committee of the Foundation Council of the College of General Practitioners recommended that all medical students should be given an insight into general practice, and that medical schools should co-opt general practitioners to advise and contribute. They concluded:

> ... we believe that an insight into the nature of general practice, and some first-hand experience of it, form an essential part of the basic training of all doctors, whatever their future may be.[1]

Throughout the 1950s and 1960s, following the creation of the College and the slow but steady establishment of university departments of general practice, attachments to general practice began to be included in many undergraduate curricula. The objectives of these courses, however, remained mainly vocational, tending not to be seen as essential to the education of doctors. Rather, they were more to do with acquainting students with the GP's work so as to inform career choice. Typically such attachments lasted between 2 and 4 weeks, and were based on an apprenticeship model. The student would observe the GP teacher while he consulted or went on home visits, undertake supervised consultations, and perhaps spend time with other members of the practice team. This was supplemented by a course of lectures and tutorials in the medical school. The fact that the learning was not usually examined formally ensured that such attachments were not taken particularly seriously by students, often being seen as light relief from an otherwise overloaded course.

A Royal Commission on medical education in 1968 recognised general practice as a distinct discipline, encouraged teaching and learning in general practice for medical students, and paved the way for the introduction of mandatory vocational training.[2] Academic general practice, and with it GP input to undergraduate courses, continued to expand through the 1970s and 1980s. There were innovations, such as the introduction of family placements and opportunities for early patient contact in the community, but these were patchy.

Despite these developments, Julian Tudor-Hart, always to be relied on for a pithy observation, was driven in his 1984 George Swift lecture to remark:

> Our system of medical education is still designed to produce community clinicians only as a by-product, an afterthought following a core curriculum designed by and for specialists. Its central aim remains for the production of specialist excellence, unsullied by prior contact with the society it serves. It is training the wrong people, at the wrong time, in the wrong skills and in the wrong place.[3]

Around the same time, a working group of the Association of University Teachers of General Practice (AUTGP) produced a report which critically appraised the General Medical Council's (GMC) 1980 recommendations on basic medical education in terms of the potential contribution general practice could make (and in some areas had been making for many years). The GMC proposed 20 educational objectives for achieving their aim that:

> by the time of qualification the graduate should have sufficient knowledge of the structure and functions of the human body in health and disease, of normal and abnormal human behaviour and of the techniques of diagnosis and treatment to enable him (sic) to assume the responsibilities of a pre-registration house officer and to prepare him for vocational training . . . [4]

The AUTGP group argued persuasively that at least 16 of the 20 objectives could not really be achieved effectively without using the educational resources of general practice. They concluded that:

> The question is not whether, but how best these resources should be used. [5]

The call for more GP teaching continued into the 1990s, [6,7] increasingly supported by evidence that general practice could not only 'come up with the goods', but that such teaching was also very highly rated by students. A new incentive for change, particularly in London, was the crisis resulting from changes in healthcare delivery, rather than any Damascene educational conversion of Deans. Reduction in the number of hospital beds and the increasing shift of care into general practice and the community meant that some medical schools were simply no longer able to provide adequate clinical experience for students in the traditional teaching hospital tertiary care setting. One response was to relocate specialist teaching, for example the traditional medical firm, in general practice, an approach pioneered by King's College Hospital Medical School. [8]

Publication of the GMC's influential document, *Tomorrow's Doctors*, in 1993 was, without doubt, a major catalyst of curriculum reform in the UK. Amongst its many recommendations (Box 4.1) there was an explicit call for more teaching and learning to take place in general practice. [9]

Box 4.1 Principal recommendations of *Tomorrow's Doctors* [9]

- Reduction of factual burden.
- Promotion of learning through curiosity.
- Inculcation of appropriate attitudes.
- Greater emphasis on acquisition of skills.
- Definition of a 'core curriculum', encouraging essential knowledge, skills, attitudes.

- Augmentation of core with a series of student-selected 'special study modules'.
- Increased emphasis on communication skills.
- Response to changing patterns of healthcare, particularly experience in the community.
- Greater emphasis on public health.
- Learning systems informed by modern educational theory.
- Establishment of effective supervisory structures.
- Introduction of appropriate methods of assessment.
- Increased prominence for ethics and the law.*
- Preparation for working in a diverse, multicultural society.*

(* These recommendations were added by the GMC in 1995)

By this time some medical schools were already running substantial community-based programmes, and most were planning to introduce more.[10] University departments of general practice were also playing a major role in the curriculum at many levels besides simple delivery of courses, including selection and admission, student support and guidance, curriculum management, and assessment. They found themselves leading curriculum development and delivery in (often vast) subject areas such as communication skills and ethics, clinical audit, evidence-based medicine, teamwork, cultural aspects of medicine and faculty development, areas previously neglected but all by now considered part of core business.

Meanwhile, throughout the 1980s another battle was being fought outside the medical schools, a struggle between academe and the mandarins of Whitehall over securing appropriate financial support for general practice teaching. The dogged persistence of several senior GP academics, in particular John Howie and John Walker, operating in sometimes Kafka-esque circumstances, led after more than a decade of frustrating negotiations to the decision to make Service Increment For Teaching (SIFT) monies (known as Additional Costs of Teaching, ACT, in Scotland), accessible to general practice. There is no doubt that the landscape of medical school curricula would look very different today without this major achievement.[11]

At the start of the millennium

Thus, at the start of the millennium, most medical schools in the UK have a significant GP component in their courses[12] with academic general practice playing a lead role in the curriculum, and perhaps a quarter of general practices nationwide involved in undergraduate teaching. In some medical schools, for example Birmingham and Liverpool, GP teaching comprises as much as 20% of curricular time. The most radical example, staged ironically in one of the most fiercely conservative institutions in the UK, was the Cambridge Community-based Clinical Course which ran between 1993 and 1998.[13] In this twin-track experiment, students spent 15 of their 27 months' clinical course based in a general practice exploring Tudor-Hart's upside-down world! The course offered students experience of both specialist and generalist education in a community setting, and was very positively evaluated.

Furthermore, pre-registration house officer (PRHO) schemes around the UK routinely offer general practice placements as part of their rotations (again, these are generally evaluated very positively). Spending time in general practice is also increasingly seen as a valid and important component of training in a growing range of specialities. Finally, it is hard to see how the planned expansion of medical student numbers (which will see an increase of over 50% nationally by the time the new programmes are fully implemented in 2003) can be achieved without significant GP and community involvement.

The shift of more basic education into the community has not been confined to the UK. The World Health Organisation has long promoted a move to more community-orientated and community-based educational programmes for health professionals. In a report in 1987[14] it gave the following six possible reasons in favour.

- Imparts a sense of social responsibility and accountability, plus an understanding of the relationship between health, illness and disease.
- Enables theory to be linked to practice.
- Breaks down the barriers between professions and the public.
- Keeps educational processes relevant by confronting reality.
- Helps the acquisition of a wide range of competencies.
- Ultimately improves the quality of community health services.

The debates about increasing teaching in general practice (or primary care) are taking place in the much broader context of the relationship between education, service and the community. What is indisputable is that the trend is global, wide-ranging and rapidly evolving. For example, a recent book on community-based education gave examples of innovations from as far afield as Africa, India, China, Scandinavia, Australia and North America, as well as the UK.[15]

So why are graduates still apparently unprepared for general practice?

With all the abovementioned changes in undergraduate education why is it that graduates are still apparently unprepared for practice?

The first, and most obvious, reason is that the effects of such developments are delayed because of the long lead time, a minimum of six years between entry to medical school and completion of the PRHO year and commencement of vocational training. Any innovation introduced today, however radical and community-oriented, will not impact for some time.

There is another more generic reason, however, which raises questions about how effective undergraduate curricula are at preparing graduates for the job of doctoring, regardless of speciality. It will be many readers' experience that they felt they learnt more about the job in the first week as a house officer than in the previous five years, and this still appears to be the case, despite the radical changes in curricula. Shifting the focus of the undergraduate course from trying to produce the all-singing, all-dancing, 'omni-competent' graduate, fit to practise autonomously on day one, to one whose aim is to produce a competent 'pluri-potential' PRHO will, again, take time to impact.

Another important factor, however, is the so-called 'hidden curriculum'.[16] A curriculum can be thought of as comprising three elements: 'the curriculum on paper' (i.e. what it is intended will be achieved); 'the curriculum in action' (i.e. what is actually delivered on the day); and 'the curriculum as experienced'. The latter can be very different from both what is intended and what actually happens. Learning that is neither explicitly intended nor formally taught is known as 'the hidden curriculum'. It is a potent force in all learning situations, and is effectively a parallel curriculum through which people pick up the values, norms and expectations of the particular setting. It still seems to be the case, certainly in the author's experience, that the generally very positive views of general practice that students gain through undergraduate attachments are slowly but surely eroded whilst working in the hospital environment. Most of this seems to come from negative views expressed by hospital colleagues, both junior and senior. Comments in feedback from students after GP placements, such as 'I hadn't realised how difficult a job general practice was; I will remember this when I am a house officer receiving admissions!', are heartening, but do not appear always to be borne out with the passage of time. It may be that, as students' attitudes towards general practice decline/deteriorate, so does their grasp of the knowledge base and orientation of the discipline.

The fourth factor relates to student selection, which is increasingly becoming a focus for reformers of medical education. Traditionally, the majority of medical school entrants in the UK are teenagers entering direct from schools in the independent sector, usually from the higher socio-economic bracket, with high academic grades in science subjects. There is evidence that certain groups have been disadvantaged in the past (including applicants from non-white ethnic minorities, older applicants, lower socio-economic groups and so on).[17] Medical students thus represent a narrow sector of society. Most have little 'life experience' and their motives for doing medicine may be unclear, often based on well-intentioned, but misguided advice from careers advisers (e.g. '...because you're good at science'). Little wonder, then, that at least some of these students do not find themselves intellectually challenged by general practice.

Part of this relates to the very nature of the discipline. Of the many differences between hospital and general practice, several stand out as potentially significant challenges to the beginning learner, or likely to induce cynicism in the student or young doctor seeking intellectual stimulation in the pursuit of 'real' diseases. One of the key distinguishing features of general practice is commitment to the person, not the disease or problem, emphasising the central importance of understanding, establishing and maintaining relationships (these 'person-patients' are also, by the by, autonomous and free-willed compared to the relatively passive and captive clientele in hospital, which poses its own particular challenges!). Other important differences include working in an environment characterised by uncertainty and complexity, using a different problem-solving strategy in which decisions are often based on minimal information, with no precedent or guidelines for action; working in relative isolation, without the familiar back-up systems of the hospital setting; the breadth (as opposed to depth) of the required knowledge base; and the fact that daily the GP is confronted not only by her successes, but also by her mistakes. In the words of John Howie, general practice:

> ... is the discipline where things are not always what they seem to be, and the way in which apparent clinical agendas and other life situations come together may be infinitely hard to determine – and not always fully understood by patients or doctors. It is the discipline where the prize for getting it right is so great and the cost of failing of such long-term consequence.'[11]

Perhaps it just takes *time* to develop the requisite competencies and attitudes to function both effectively and happily in general practice, more time than may be available in even a prolonged GP attachment; and perhaps learning the ropes can only take place 'on the job'.

The final reason for young doctors' apparent lack of preparedness for general practice is that curricula, on the whole, tend to be focused more on producing doctors for practice in *today's* circumstances, rather than practising in tomorrow's world. In the words of one set of authors:

> ... professional education often reflects the needs of a past situation, serving the professional claims and values which were the basis of an earlier system and which sustained the original claims to professional legitimacy'.[15]

Thus areas such as management, clinical governance, teamwork and leadership, all pertinent to the work of the 'new GP',[18] are only just beginning to be addressed in undergraduate curricula. Of course, it is impossible to predict precisely what kind of medicine tomorrow's doctors will be practising, and how. We can only be certain that it will be different, and that continuing change is the order of the day.

What *can* learning in the community and general practice bring to medical education (and what is the evidence?)

The view of the College founding fathers that experience in general practice as an undergraduate was essential for all, regardless of career intentions, was visionary and has been vindicated over and over again as it has become apparent just what general practice can offer medical education. Box 4.2 lists some of the areas of learning to which general practice can make an important contribution, many supported by a growing evidence base. Many of them, of course, can (and should) be achieved in both hospital and community settings, but several are probably better or can only be achieved in general practice. Some of these are discussed in more detail below.

Box 4.2 What can learning in the community and general practice offer medical education?

- 'Common things are common'.*
- Management of 'undifferentiated' problems.*
- Early presentation, and evolution of disease and illness.*
- Conditions rarely seen in hospital.*
- Early patient contact.
- Development of professional skills and attitudes.

- Tolerance of uncertainty and ambiguity.
- Integration of knowledge (basic science/clinical science, and across disciplines).
- Aspects of population medicine.*
- Development of an holistic approach to clinical practice.
- Longitudinal aspects of care, including continuity.*
- Environmental and social determinants of disease.*
- Health, illness and disability in its social context.*
- Organisational and other key features of general practice (e.g. primary/secondary acre interface, and the gatekeeper role).*
- General practice as a career, and the 'life and times' of practitioners.*
- Social awareness and responsibility.
- A positive learning environment.
- Good role models.

(* Asterisked areas are those which may be best or can only be learnt in general practice and community settings)

- *'Common things are common'* is an age-old pearl of wisdom beloved of medical teachers, but so much the case that, generally speaking, in most clinical settings, uncommon presentations of *common* conditions are still more common than common presentations of *uncommon* problems! Exposure to the wide range of (common) problems seen in general practice, at all stages from presentation as an '*undifferentiated*' problem through to resolution, chronicity or otherwise, will help students develop clinical reasoning skills. General practice placements have been shown to expose students to a wide range of relevant problems.[19]
- Engaging with real patients at an early stage provides a powerful motivational context for learning, increases understanding of the role of the doctor and the nature of the doctor–patient relationship, and may promote the development of empathy. General practice has been shown to provide an ideal setting for *early patient contact* with junior medical students.[20]
- General practice also provides an excellent location for the acquisition of professional skills. Students not only have access to an appropriate number and variety of patients,[21] they also acquire their *clinical skills* just as well, if not better, than in hospital.[22] Historically, general practice educators have led the way with teaching *communication skills*, and these

successes have been transferred to the undergraduate setting, promoting a more patient-centred approach.[13,23]

- Learning medicine in the community offers opportunities not easily found in hospital. For example, *health, illness and disability* can be studied in their social (i.e. natural) context, as can the *environmental and social determinants of health and disease.*[24] This may help develop a more *holistic approach*, seeing patients as people rather than dysfunctional machines, as well as an appreciation of the *uncertainties and ambiguities* that lie at the heart of medical practice.

- During a GP placement, students will of course see a wide range of *clinical conditions not seen, or rarely seen, in hospital* (except when serious complications have developed). Common childhood infections, shingles, polymyalgia, skin infections, problems of the climacteric, insomnia, acute gout, tendinitis, influenza, anxiety and depression, migraine, mechanical back pain, contraception ... the list goes on. Areas of practice which may be best seen in general practice include the gatekeeper role and other aspects of the primary–secondary care interface, long-term management of chronic diseases, childhood immunisation and other preventive strategies, and the aftermath of surgery, to name a few. Of course there are specific issues that can *only* be appreciated in practice, for example *general practice as a career* and *organisational aspects of practice.*

- One of the most important features of the Cambridge experiment was the opportunity students had to establish and maintain long-term relationships with patients, in contrast to the usual compartmentalisation and lack of continuity of traditional courses. Students found this a valuable and important feature of the programme, and again, the experience may have helped develop a more *holistic approach.*[13]

- GP attachments generally receive very positive feedback from students. Comments such as 'this was the best attachment at medical school' are not uncommon in the author's experience. Apart from the content of attachments, however, many of the favourable things that students say relate to the positive learning environment and the quality of tutoring, for example enthusiastic teachers, feeling valued, timely feedback, doing rather than observing, and so on.[25,26] GP teachers also make *good role models.* One challenge for curriculum planners and those involved in faculty development is to transfer some of these attributes to the hospital environment.

The long and short of this growing body of evidence is that we can teach more or less anything we wish to in the general practice setting, other than the obvious 'high tech' and 'fire engine' medicine. The real question is what is taught best in what setting, and by whom?

The impacts of teaching in general practice

At the outset of the recent expansion in general practice teaching, caution was expressed about the possible impacts on practice, and the ability of GPs and the service to implement and sustain high quality teaching programmes. For example, Higgs and Jones highlighted several areas in which such teaching could have a negative impact, including on quality of care and the doctor–patient relationship (arguing that the traditional GP consultation is private, with a doctor known to the patient, and does not normally include a third party), continuity of care and practice organisation (for example, effects on space, time and productivity).[27] Concern was also expressed about the resource implications of the proposed expansions.[28] Commentators on this issue have been unanimous in their contention that general practice teaching will only succeed, and be sustainable, if it is adequately resourced and rewarded.

What has been the impact so far of increasing teaching in general practice? Without doubt teaching has a significant impact on many aspects of practice organisation – although the problems are not insurmountable – requiring at the very least careful planning and timetabling, and for major involvement the provision of dedicated space, extra practice staff and other learning resources.

Several studies have shown that teaching students can have a positive effect on the morale of GP teachers, along with other perceived benefits such as improvements in clinical skills and knowledge, beneficial changes in clinical practice and practice organisation, a positive effect on 'team spirit' and, for practices, a better public image. On the whole, the benefits seem to outweigh the disadvantages.[29,30]

Patients generally react positively towards the presence of students in the surgery. Most seem only too pleased to help, often seeing participation as an opportunity for 'payback' to the health system, and their main concerns are around consent and confidentiality. Besides this there is little published work on the benefits or disadvantages to patients of involvement in teaching, other than increased satisfaction and feeling better informed as a result.[31]

However, evidence is accumulating that increased exposure to primary and community care influences career intentions of undergraduates, enhances their views of the role of primary care within the health service and may promote holistic attitudes.[32,33]

Clearly more evidence is required about the impact of GP teaching at all levels. Researching such a complex area presents considerable methodological challenges.

Educating tomorrow's GPs

It is recognised that medical education at all levels will need to change to meet new challenges, and to prepare adaptable practitioners, regardless of their chosen career path. As George Silver said:

> Medical education is a reflection of medical practice; it is not education that will change the practitioners, but reformed practice that will redesign medical education.[3]

What are these challenges? A number of major trends that will influence the medicine of tomorrow are already in full flow. These include, in no particular order:

- changes in demography (for example, the increasing proportion of elderly people and the growth in displaced, migrant populations)
- advances in our understanding about the biology of health and disease, and our ability to intervene, against a background of finite resources
- the ethical implications of these advances and resource constraints
- the information explosion, and the revolution in communications and information technology
- changing patterns of healthcare delivery (in the context of this chapter, notably the shift of care into the community).

Another major force is the changing expectations of, and demands for, healthcare from both the public and politicians. The traditional paternalistic role of the doctor is outmoded, and what society wants from us includes: greater accountability; partnership; improved attitudes and better communication; better quality of information; more choice; technically competent care; and advocacy. Doctors are expected to respect and protect all patients, keep up to date, and demonstrate high ethical and moral standards.[34]

The nature and content of general practice is also changing. A debate about the role of the general practitioner rumbled on throughout the 1990s, precipitated by the major health reforms of that decade. This was taking place in the context of a wider debate about the role of medicine and the core values of the profession, and the need for medical schools to redefine their mission (i.e. to become less remote from the communities they serve). Other contextual factors included: the increasing autonomy (and threat!) of nursing and allied health professionals; changes in the organisation and delivery of primary care (such as the establishment of primary care groups and trusts, remodelling of the contractual status of GPs, the creation of *NHS Direct* and so on); the introduction of clinical governance; and the recruitment crisis. The importance of the role of clinical generalist is a key theme in this debate,[35] as is the need for a new definition for general practice.[36,37]

Finally, highly pertinent to the problems of recruitment and retention, there are the changes in the attitudes and aspirations of the younger generations entering and graduating from medical school. They want a 'life', a more humane balance between home and work, and will demand training, support, career options and flexibility (*see* Chapter 1).

All these have major implications for medical education, both at under-graduate and postgraduate levels.

What are the competencies required of tomorrow's practitioners? Much has been written about the requirements to function effectively in this brave new world. Some suggestions are shown in Box 4.3. Of course most of these are desirable attributes for *any* practitioner, regardless of speciality.

Box 4.3 Some competencies and attributes of tomorrow's practitioners

- Take responsibility for own learning.
- Manage information.
- Be flexible and self-aware.
- Have critical reasoning skills.
- Be able to work in a team.
- Show leadership skills.
- Be a good communicator.
- Show ethical awareness and reasoning skills.
- Participate in a culturally diverse society.
- Provide cost-effective and appropriate care.
- Promote healthy lifestyles.

Undergraduate curricula are already tackling many of these areas, guided by *Tomorrow's Doctors* and other policy documents. Most medical schools now include strands on personal and professional development (PPD) as part of their core curriculum. For example, in the new curriculum at the Universi-ties of Newcastle and Durham (Stockton Campus), a PPD strand occupies around one-sixth of curricular time and covers a wide range of areas such as communication skills, ethics, informatics, cultural diversity, evidence-based practice, study methods and 'self-care'. It is integrated with other learning and is fully assessed.

New educational approaches are now widespread. These include greater integration (both horizontal and vertical), outcome-based education, problem-based learning, more appropriate assessment methods, interprofessional learning, promotion of reflective practice, broadening of experience through the introduction of special study modules, a greater role for humanities (*see* Chapter 5) and so on. Student selection is being addressed in a number of ways so as to widen access to medical school, such as lowering the threshold of academic grades and dropping mandatory science subjects, backed up by specific outreach programmes in schools to attract students with 'non-traditional' backgrounds. Several medical schools now offer graduate entry programmes.

It has to be said that many of these new strategies, whilst having powerful intuitive appeal and major political backing, are not supported (as yet) by evidence in favour, for example multiprofessional learning, changes to student selection procedures, introduction of more student choice. Clearly much evaluation and research is needed.

Meanwhile, arguments have been made for the creation of medical schools whose specific purpose is to train doctors for work in the community.[38] This is a controversial notion, and for the time being the main focus of undergraduate curricula in the UK is likely to remain the production of a competent PRHO ready to embark on higher professional training whatever their chosen speciality. That general practice will play a major part in the process is beyond doubt.[39]

The increase in GP and community-based teaching poses many potential challenges.[40] Some of these are shown in Box 4.4.

Box 4.4 Challenges of increased teaching in general practice and the community

- Capacity.
- Resources.
- Impact (organisation, productivity, patients).
- Quality control.
- Teacher training and support.
- 'Burn out'.
- Relationship between academe and service.
- Research and evaluation.

(Adapted from Murray E and Modell M (1999) Community-based teaching: the challenges. *BJGPP*. **49**: 395–8)

As discussed previously, most of these can be tackled with sufficient vision and creativity, strong institutional support and, of course, adequate resourcing. Community-based teaching is not a cheap option. Capacity remains the biggest unknown factor, particularly in the long term. Will there be enough teaching practices to support the proposed increases in undergraduate, PRHO and SHO placements, in addition to new developments such as interprofessional learning, as service demands on general practice and on GPs continue to grow, and recruitment and retention remain an issue?

Thus far the situation seems to be manageable and one may be cautiously optimistic; in the experience of the author (and others) there is a pool of enthusiastic and skilled teachers in suitable practices to support a realistic expansion. Furthermore, the NHS is taking more of an interest in the education and training of its workforce, and models for integrating teaching and learning, personal and professional development, and service delivery in primary care are being described.[41]

Conclusion

In this chapter I have put undergraduate teaching in general practice in an historical context up to the present day, when it is playing a major part in UK curricula. I explored some of the reasons why, despite these developments, entrants to general practice still appear to be unprepared for the job. What general practice can offer to undergraduate education is then discussed (just about anything we want!), along with some of the impacts of moving more teaching and learning into the community. The chapter ends with a reflection on the competencies required of 'tomorrow's doctors' and how general practice is playing, and will continue to play, a significant role in their education.

Summary

- General practitioners increasingly teach tomorrow's doctors.
- Learning in the community benefits all, not least future hospital specialists.
- Although enthusiastic during student attachments, many young doctors reject general practice as a career option.

References

1   Barber GO *et al.* (1953) The teaching of general practice by general practitioners. *BMJ.* **4 July**: 36–8.

2   Todd Report (1968) *Report of the Royal Commission on Medical Education.* Cmnd 3569. HMSO: London.

3   Hart JT (1985) The world turned upside down: proposals for community-based undergraduate medical education. *JRCGP.* **35**: 63–8.

4   General Medical Council (1980) *Recommendations on Basic Medical Education.* GMC, London.

5   Association of University Teachers of General Practice, United Kingdom & Republic of Ireland (1984) *Undergraduate medical education in general practice. Occasional Paper 28.* Royal College of General Practitioners, London.

6   Oswald N (1991) Where should we train doctors in the future? Less in hospitals, more in general practices. *BMJ.* **303**: 71.

7   Towle A (1991) *Critical Thinking: the future of undergraduate medical education.* King's Fund, London.

8   Seabrook M, Booton P and Evans T (1994) *Widening the Horizons of Medical Education.* King's Fund, London.

9   General Medical Council (1993) *Tomorrow's Doctors. Recommendations on undergraduate medical education.* GMC, London.

10   Robinson LA, Spencer JA and Jones RH (2001) Contribution of academic departments of general practice to undergraduate teaching, and their plans for curriculum development. *British Journal of General Practice.* **44**: 489–91.

11   Howie J (1999) *Patient-centredness and the Politics of Change. A day in the life of academic general practice.* Nuffield Trust, London.

12   Association for the Study of Medical Education (1997) *Curriculum Innovations: descriptions of undergraduate medical courses in the UK* (conference papers). ASME, Edinburgh.

13   Oswald N, Alderson T and Jones S (2001) Evaluating primary care as a base for medical education: the report of the Cambridge Community-based Clinical Course. *Medical Education.* **35**: 782–8.

14   World Health Organisation (1987) *Technical report series no 746. Community-based education of health personnel. Report of a WHO study group.* WHO, Geneva.

15   Boaden N and Bligh J (1999) *Community-based Medical Education. Towards a shared agenda for learning.* Arnold, London.

16   Snyder BR (1971) *The Hidden Curriculum.* Knopf, New York.

17   Wood DF (1999) Medical school selection – fair or unfair? *Medical Education.* **33**: 399–401.

18   Harrison J, Innes R and van Zwanenberg T (eds) (2001) *The New GP: changing roles and the modern NHS.* Radcliffe Medical Press, Oxford.

19   Alderson TStJ and Oswald NT (1999) Clinical experience of medical students in primary care: use of an electronic log in monitoring experience and in

guiding education in the Cambridge Community Based Clinical Course. *Medical Education.* **33**: 429–33.

20   Hampshire AJ (1998) Providing early clinical experience in primary care. *Medical Education.* **32**: 495–501.

21   Parle JV, Greenfield SM, Skelton J, Lester H and Hobbs FDR (1997) Acquisition of basic clinical skills in the general practice setting. *Medical Education.* **31**: 99–104.

22   Murray E, Jolly B and Modell M (1997) Can students learn clinical method in general practice? A randomized crossover trial based on objective structured clinical examinations. *BMJ.* **315**: 920–3.

23   Thistlethwaite JE and Jordan JJ (1999) Patient-centred consultations: a comparison of student experience and understanding in two clinical environments. *Medical Education.* **33**: 678–85.

24   Whitehouse CR (1998) The community experience in the new Manchester medical undergraduate curriculum: reactions to the first module. *Education for Health.* **11**: 173–82.

25   Snadden D and Yaphe J (1996) General practice and medical education: what do medical students value? *Medical Teacher.* **18**: 31–4.

26   Foldevi M (1995) Undergraduate medical students' ratings of a clerkship in general practice. *Family Practice.* **12**: 207–13.

27   Higgs R and Jones R (1995) The impacts of increased general practice teaching in the undergraduate medical curriculum. *Education for General Practice.* **6**: 218–25.

28   Spencer J, Robinson AL, Corradine A and Smith D (1997) Evaluation of the impact of clinical skills teaching on general practice. In: AJ Scherpbier *et al. Advances in Medical Education.* Kluwer, London, pp. 299–301.

29   Hartley S, Macfarlane F, Gantley M and Murray E (1999) Influence on general practitioners of teaching undergraduates: qualitative study of London general practitioner teachers. *BMJ.* **319**: 1168–71.

30   Wilson A, Fraser R, McKinley RK, Preston-Whyte E and Wynn A (1996) Undergraduate teaching in the community: can general practice deliver? *British Journal of General Practice.* **46**: 45–60.

31   Spencer J, Blackmore D, Heard S *et al.* (2000) Patient-oriented learning: a review of the role of the patient in the education of medical students. *Medical Education.* **34**: 851–7.

32   Sullivan F and Morrison J (1997) What can universities do to reverse the decline in numbers of doctors entering general practice? *Medical Education.* **31**: 235–6.

33   Howe A and Ives G (2001) Does community-based experience alter career preference? New evidence from a prospective longitudinal cohort study of undergraduate medical students. *Medical Education.* **35**: 392–7.

34   General Medical Council (1998) *Good Medical Practice.* GMC, London.

35   Royal College of General Practitioners (1996) *The Nature of General Practice. Report from general practice number 37.* RCGP, London.

36   Lipman T (2000) The future general practitioner: out of date and running out of time. *British Journal of General Practice.* **50**: 743–6.

37 Olesen F, Dickinson J and Hjortdahl P (2000) General practice – time for a new definition. *BMJ*. **320**: 354–7.

38 Bligh J (1999) Is it time for a community-based medical school in the UK? *Medical Education*. **33**: 315.

39 Worley P, March R and Worley E (2000) Scanning the horizon of training for general practice. *Medical Teacher*. **22**: 452–4.

40 Murray E and Modell M (1999) Community-based teaching: the challenges. *British Journal of General Practice*. **49**: 395–8.

41 Howe A (2000) Primary care education for the new NHS: a discussion paper. *Medical Education*. **34**: 385–90.

CHAPTER 5

Arts and humanities in medical education

Jane Macnaughton

He carried ... the conviction that the medical profession as it might be was the finest in the world; presenting the most perfect interchange between science and art; offering the most perfect alliance between intellectual conquest and the social good.
George Elliot on Lydgate in *Middlemarch*

This chapter describes the link between the medical humanities and the arts and health movement, and explores their role in medical education. A number of existing courses point the way for the future.

Introduction

Recent changes in thinking on undergraduate medical education have led to an increasing emphasis on the development of doctors who know how to use and access up-to-date knowledge rather than on doctors who know a lot.[1] This is appropriate in an age when medical knowledge is under continual review. At the same time as giving thought to the development of the good technical doctor, educationalists are also turning their minds to what makes good humane practitioners – and how to educate them. It is here that the arts and humanities are beginning to make a contribution to the extent that it is not an exaggeration to speak of the medical humanities 'movement' in medical education. At the same time there has grown up in healthcare circles an awareness of what the arts can contribute to therapy and to improving the deprived environment, an important determinant of ill health. This awareness has issued in a second movement, often called the 'arts and health movement'.

Arts and health and medical humanities: why now?

There seems to have been an epidemic of arts and humanities courses breaking out in medical schools all over the country. Newcastle, Nottingham, the Royal Free and University College London, Guy's, King's and St Thomas', Aberdeen, Cardiff, Leeds and others are running special study modules for students with titles such as 'Poetry, Novels and Medicine' (Newcastle) and 'Visualising/Modifying the Body in Art and Medicine' (Guy's, King's and St Thomas'). These courses are proving very popular and there is competition for students to do them. There is also growing interest in the humanities in postgraduate medical education. A course has been run in Ripon for general practice trainers to encourage them to use the arts and humanities in the training of their GP registrars (personal communication from Dr Elaine Powey) and the Swansea MA in Medical Humanities is now well established.

In tandem with these developments in medical education is the growth of interest and activity in the arts as therapy. There are two kinds of ways in which the arts are being used for therapeutic purposes. Firstly, there are the arts therapies where visual art, music, dance and creative writing are being used by specifically trained practitioners working with groups or individuals who have an illness or disability. Music and art therapy are officially recognised as professions allied to medicine and have professional status and a recognised training.[2] The second way in which the arts are being used is for community development and health. In this context health promoters, local arts organisations and individual artists are working not in healthcare contexts with people who are ill but with communities or groups within communities which have high deprivation and are regarded as socially excluded. It is this group of activities which has helped to thrust the arts and health movement into the limelight, as social exclusion is now regarded as a major determinant of ill health[3] and is recognised as such by the government, who are interested in anything that may contribute to tackling it.[4] There is, therefore, a political imperative to encourage the development of community arts and health projects and the government has even made mention of the importance of these activities in the recent white paper on health, *Saving Lives: our healthier nation*, commenting that:

participation in the arts and sport can promote social cohesion by building strong social networks.[5]

Medical humanities and arts and health: a relationship

The two movements are related as they both deal with applications of the arts in health and medicine, but there are differences. Firstly, the arts and health movement is dedicated to improving the health of individuals or communities whereas the medical humanities movement is concerned with the educational development of the health practitioner and with the critical examination of the nature of healthcare and medical practice and its evidence base.[6] The former movement is a community and health-related activity, while the latter is a professional development and educational activity which has grown up within universities, largely within medical schools. The origins of both movements can, however, be traced to some common roots: changing views of the determinants of health; and related changes in society's view of biomedical medicine and of doctors who practise it. Let us examine these common roots.

The current New Labour government in the UK has explicitly acknowledged the fact that 'the social, economic and environmental factors tending towards poor health are potent' and that inequalities in health between richer and poorer is a widespread problem.[7] This acceptance has committed the government and the health services to examine ways of tackling the determinants of health inequalities. Until now the NHS has focused its attention on tackling the health of the individual but, as Richard Wilkinson says in his seminal book on the social determinants of health:

> ... the important factors which make some societies healthier than others may be quite different from those which differ between healthy and unhealthy individuals within the same society.[8]

Those important factors, according to Wilkinson, include the extent of economic and social equality within the society, and the extent to which people feel they have control over their lives. The problem is not so much to do with absolute levels of poverty but rather to do with the extent to which there are large gradients between the 'haves' and the 'have nots'. These issues are not ones which we would expect to be the concern of health services. Rather they are the concern of governments and welfare agencies. But to the extent to which they are now being recognised as important for health, doctors must be aware of the problem of societal inequality and consider ways of tackling the lack of control that it produces.

This new social economic view of the origins of health problems is a challenge to the pervasive biomedical approach to medicine in the UK and most Western societies. It is a challenge to doctors to promote a new way of working and, in consequence, to encourage a change to the way in which future doctors are educated. The arts and health movement is responding to this changing view by using the arts to promote greater social cohesion and involvement. There is evidence that community arts and health projects are having this effect. A recent report published by the independent research organisation Comedia found that participation in the arts can increase people's confidence and sense of self-worth, extend involvement in social activity and encourage adults to take up education and training experiences.[9] Granted, then, that there is hard evidence that the arts can promote health in communities, what is now required from doctors and from doctors in training is an awareness of this important health determinant. Doctors must acquire a broader conceptual understanding of the basis of health inequalities and how these cause ill health. In turn this should encourage doctors to develop a bigger conceptual toolkit for tackling health problems.

This brings us back to the connection between arts and health and medical humanities. The arts and health movement is a response to the need to tackle social exclusion through community involvement with the arts. The medical humanities movement may be seen as an attempt to extend the range of doctors beyond biomedicine in two ways. Firstly, by extending the scope of medical education beyond biomedicine doctors can be given access to a whole new range of concepts for understanding the variety of contexts in which health-improving activities can take place, the varied types of evidence relevant to different aspects of the medical consultation, and indeed for understanding health itself in its varied meaning for different people. Secondly, the traditional and rapidly expanding technical expertise of biomedicine can be given a humane basis.

A humane basis: the educational context

As well as having a relationship to the parallel arts and health movement, the medical humanities movement has arisen against the background of changes in the educational context. In the past, ethics was the subject that both brought humanities back into the context of medical education and also brought academics such as philosophers and theologians into medical education. But now, as part of the need to widen the basis for medical expertise, there is a move to suggest that the teaching of ethics is too narrow a field to take in the range of moral and personal difficulties that may affect clinical decision making. This point is taken up by Robin Downie in the *Journal of Medical Ethics*.[10] In a commentary on a poem, Downie argues that most of what has been traditionally taught via undergraduate courses on medical ethics can be taught in the richer context of the medical humanities. This richer context can provide a wide non-medical perspective on problems in medical ethics and assist with the 'consciousness-raising' aspects of ethics. The point here is while medical ethics tends to concentrate on what are called 'dilemmas', many of the criticisms of doctors derive from the fact that they have a manner which patients find arrogant, or they can write letters unaware of the impact these might have on their patients. The humanities can hold up a mirror to ourselves, which the more theoretical approach of philosophical medical ethics cannot do. It may be that the umbrella discipline for ethics in the future may be medical humanities, which will allow the fuller consideration of all these qualities in the developing doctor.

The expansion in the number of medical schools and the need to train more doctors is also having an effect on admissions criteria. Wider access to prospective students who have been educated in other disciplines, including the arts, is being encouraged. Teaching methods within medical schools are diversifying from the standard method of information-giving in large group lectures to increasing focus on small group teaching and problem-based learning. These encourage the students to think for themselves and to be more critically aware of what they are being taught: very much the attributes of the humanely educated arts student.

Above all, the undergraduate medical educational context has changed through the efforts of the General Medical Council. In 1993 they recognised that medical education needed a radical rethink and, in their document *Tomorrow's Doctors*,[11] recommended a greater focus on education, as opposed to training, in the undergraduate degree. The good doctor, as the GMC suggests, must be an educated doctor and this is one of the major areas where arts and humanities subjects might make a contribution.[12]

Helping doctors cope

Working in the caring professions is hard. It involves contact with blood, sweat and tears – and worse. It also frequently requires doctors to hear of others' distress, both physical and psychological. Patients and clients invest a great deal in doctors and expect much. Often they expect more than doctors are able to deliver and this results in disappointment and sometimes anger. It seems that doctors are finding it more and more difficult to deal with the pressures. A study in 1993 of job satisfaction among British GPs indicated that GPs were becoming less happy with their lot than they had been in 1987 and that the male doctors in particular had significantly higher levels of anxiety and depression than the population norm.[13] The main predictors of anxiety and depression were the job stressors associated with the demands of the job and patients' expectations. When doctors and other health professionals get 'burnout' – the currently fashionable term – there is a move towards what is called 'depersonalisation' of the patient.[14] This is a protective mechanism designed to shield the doctor from the need to respond in a human way to the patient and to take their cares and concerns on.

It is, therefore, a damaging experience for doctor and patient alike when the job gets too much. We have a responsibility to develop individuals who are equipped to deal with the pain and distress patients may bring to them. Most of the young people entering medicine will not have had personal experiences to draw on which will help them identify with their patients, but surely this is not required. A study carried out at the University of Newcastle, NSW, showed that the graduates from their non-traditional programme, which took in undergraduates from arts as well as science backgrounds, were more likely to experience greater quality of life in their future careers than those who had been to more traditional schools.[15] The investigators concluded that the GPs from the non-traditional school may have had more realistic expectations about life in clinical practice and also they may have had greater capacity to respond to the needs of the patients because of the breadth of their educational experience. What the arts can help develop in doctors is the imaginative insight which will engage their active concern in dealing with patients. What do I mean by this?

Those writing on medical education or communication skills often speak of the importance of 'empathy'. But this concept may put the emphasis on the wrong place. The focus should not be on the doctor's own feelings in response to the patient, but on the patient's problem and what to do about it. Downie draws a helpful analogy here with a musician:

> The performer's attention is not inward – he'd lose the place if he was looking inward – but outwards towards the music. The feeling, as it were, is in the fingers. Similarly, the doctor's attention should be outward towards the patient, and his feeling with, or his compassion for, the patient should be shown in an imaginative grasp of the patient's whole situation.[16]

This brings us to imagination. Imagination involves a conscious grasp or understanding of another's situation. Whereas empathy is an instinctive reaction to another's distress – and we all have this capacity to a greater or lesser extent – imagination has a cognitive aspect. This point is illustrated by the following passage from a book called *A Fortunate Man* by John Berger. This is the story of a country doctor whose life and work is observed and analysed by Berger with great sensitivity and insight. In this passage, the doctor (whose name is Sassall) goes though a kind of crisis of understanding himself and his patients. Until this time he prided himself mainly on his ability to deal with saving lives and has little patience with the less clearly medical problems in his patients' lives:

> After a few years he began to change. He was in his mid-thirties: at that time of life when, instead of being spontaneously oneself, as in one's twenties, it is necessary, in order to remain honest, to confront oneself and judge from a second position ... He became aware of the possibility of his patients changing. They, as they became more used to him, sometimes made confessions for which there was no medical reference so far as he had learnt. He began to take a different view of the meaning of the term crisis ... He began to realise that he must face his imagination, even explore it. It must no longer lead always to the 'unimaginable' ... to his contemplating only fights within the jaws of death ... He began to realise that imagination had to be lived with on every level: his own imagination first – because otherwise this could distort his observation – and then the imagination of his patients.[17]

These observations by Berger reflect the experience of many doctors. There is a period of intense activity in their twenties when young doctors are going through specialist training and long stretches on call. This is a time when most people are finding out about themselves and learning more about what makes them tick. Young doctors in training miss out on this. They then emerge in their early to mid-thirties having attained the hoped-for goal and find themselves wondering what it was all about, who they are and, in particular, how can they relate as people to the patients they are trying to treat. This point returns us to the importance of educational initiative in protecting doctors from burnout. Doctors need to develop those aspects of themselves as human beings that will enable them to recognise other people in their humanity and distress, not just in order to feel sympathy but to become engaged actively in helping. Chief amongst these attributes (as Berger describes) is imagination. What better teacher of the imagination than the works of great creative imaginations themselves: novels, plays and poems.

Practicalities: undergraduate and postgraduate education

One model for humanities teaching is that students should simply attend a course in an arts faculty. This model, which David Greaves calls 'additive',[18] has the advantages of introducing medical students to non-medical ways of looking at the world, non-medical ways of teaching and non-medical students. This model recommends itself as having the greatest educational merit of the three models I will describe, but it has an almost overwhelming disadvantage in that teaching in another faculty is difficult to arrange and medical students may not make the connections with medical practice (if that matters).

A second model, preferred by Greaves, he calls 'integrative'. Courses offered in terms of this model would put medical knowledge in a wider perspective. A good example of the integrative model in practice is 'Ethics in Medicine' which is run as a compulsory course at the University of Aberdeen.[19] This course includes the following amongst its core aims:

> To demonstrate that the resolution of ethical dilemmas in medical practice can be assisted by rational analysis, including the use of philosophical techniques.
>
> To introduce the concept that much learning, relevant to ethical dilemmas in medicine, can be gained from the study of various forms of the Arts and Humanities about why moral stances are taken by society and individuals.

There are as yet few examples in practice of the humanities as integrative but it is likely to be a growth area in medical education in the next few years.

A third model (not mentioned by Greaves) might be called the 'complementary'. The aim of courses offered in this model would be to broaden students' awareness of other conceptual approaches and to extend their imaginations. Such courses depend on the student's ability to follow Forster's mantra 'only connect'.[20] John Berger's country doctor, Sassall, demonstrated his ability to make these imaginative connections in the book *A Fortunate Man*,[21] to which I have already referred. Sassall is described as 'much influenced by the books of Conrad' and had been resolved as a child to become a sailor rather than a doctor. In this passage Berger described Sassall changing in his approach to medicine through making a connection with the experience of Conrad's Master Mariners:

> He began to realise that the way Conrad's Master Mariners came to terms with their imagination – denying it any expression but projecting it all on to the sea which they then faced as though it were simultaneously their personal justification and their personal enemy – was not suitable for a doctor in his position. He had done just that – using illness and medical dangers as they used the sea. He begin to realise that he must face his imagination, even explore it. It must no longer always lead to the 'unimaginable', as it had with the Master Mariners contemplating the possible fury of the elements – or, as in his case, to his contemplating only fights within the jaws of death itself. (The clichés are essential to the vision.) He began to realise that imagination had to be lived with on every level: his own imagination first – because otherwise this could distort his observation – and then the imagination of his patients.[22]

In this complementary model the humanities can be seen as holding up a mirror to the medical view of the world to encourage students to make comparisons, see similarities and be challenged by differences. One example of a special study module which attempts to do this is one on political philosophy at Glasgow University.[23] In this module students read the entire text of Plato's *Republic* and attend lectures in the philosophy department. The seminar discussions are based on themes dealt with in the *Republic* which have particular relevance to the students at this point in their course (second year). One theme is 'The Family' and at this time the students are halfway through their Family Project, which involves them in a number of visits to a family and reflection on the function of families in society. They are able to contrast Plato's radical view that the family should be abolished with the view of our society (and also of the current government) that the family is the backbone of society and provides its stability. The students are, therefore, led to challenge and question these prevailing views, and they commented in the evaluation that the module had taught them to question their own views more. Unlike the integrative model, the complementary model does not pretend to provide a structure for understanding the rest of the course, but it may give students a methodology for analysing other problems and remind them of the importance of wider cultural awareness.

Practicalities: the postgraduate scene

With the introduction of a freer curriculum structure than the traditional and of Special Study Modules, there are great opportunities for arts and humanities subjects to be studied by medical students. What, however, of the opportunities for practising doctors, specifically GPs? There is great interest in this amongst GPs who recognise the need to diversify their postgraduate educational opportunities for the reasons discussed above: to help widen their imaginative approach to dealing with their patients. One course in which I was recently involved had been set up by a GP trainer, who had herself experienced the benefits of the arts in their broadest sense in her work as a practitioner and as a trainer of young GPs. I joined her for a two-day course for GP trainers to discuss how they could use the arts in their own work and, in particular, how they could encourage this in their GP registrars. We discussed music, dance, drama and, of course, literature. One of the most interesting sessions was music. The GP trainers were encouraged to bring along music which meant something to them or which they found soothing. One GP found listening to Bach helpful to sort out his thoughts prior to seeing patients about bad news. Another found the songs of Schubert gave him a deeper understanding of heartbreak and love.

Such courses and ideas in the postgraduate arena are at an early stage of development but there is interest and enthusiasm for this approach.

Conclusion

The three structural models for the application of medical humanities in medical schools are all currently being used. The most common is the third model, the complementary, but the second, the integrative, is becoming more important. The first model, the additive, is the only one of the three which might be described as 'non-instrumental' in its relationship to the development of students as doctors. All three models for the humanities will assist the students in developing the wider toolkit of concepts and approaches to the practice of medicine which is now necessary for tackling the social determinants of health, which are of increasing importance in developed societies in the twenty-first century.

Summary

- Arts and humanities have a contribution to make both in improving health and in educating doctors.
- Doctors in training may be deprived of important formative experiences derived from the arts.
- Developing doctors' imagination may help them to understand patients better *and* avoid their own burnout.

References

1   General Medical Council (1993) *Tomorrow's Doctors: recommendations on under-graduate medical education.* GMC, London.
2   Music therapy was granted professional status in 1999 through the Council for Professions Supplementary to Medicine (CPSM).
3   Wilkinson RG (1996) *Unhealthy Societies: the afflictions of inequality.* Routledge, London.
4   Social Exclusion Unit (2000) *National Strategy for Neighbourhood Renewal: a framework for consultation.* Cabinet Office, London.
5   Department of Health (1999) *Saving Lives: our healthier nation.* HMSO, London.
6   Downie RS and Macnaughton J (2000) *Clinical Judgement: evidence in practice.* Oxford University Press, Oxford.
7   Department of Health *op. cit.*, Executive Summary p.2.
8   Wilkinson *op. cit.*, p.1.
9   Matarasso F (1997) *Use or Ornament? The social impact of participation in the arts.* Comedia, London.
10 Downie RS (1999) The role of literature in medical education. A commentary on the poem: Roswell, Hanger 84. *Journal of Medical Ethics.* **25**: 529–31.
11 General Medical Council, *op. cit.*
12 Downie (1999) *op. cit.*
13 Sutherland VJ and Cooper CL (1993) Identifying distress among general practitioners: predictors of psychological ill-health and job dissatisfaction. *Social Science and Medicine.* **37**(5): 578–81.
14 Kirwan M and Armstrong D (1995) Investigation of burnout in a sample of British general practitioners. *British Journal of General Practice.* **45**(394): 259–60.
15 Hazell P, Pearson S-A and Rolfe I (1996) Influences on the quality of life of general practitioners in New South Wales, Australia. *Education for Health.* **9**: 229–37.
16 Downie RS (2001). In: M Evans and I Finlay (eds) *Medical Humanities.* BMJ Books, London.
17 Berger J (1997) *A Fortunate Man.* Vintage International, New York.
18 Evans M and Finlay I (2001) *Medical Humanities.* BMJ Books, London.
19 See 'Learning Guide to the Ethics in Medicine Special Study Module', University of Aberdeen, 1999. Course co-ordinator is Dr Ross Taylor.
20 Forster EM (1969) *Howard's End.* Penguin Books, Harmondsworth.
21 Berger *op. cit.*
22 Berger *op. cit.*
23 Downie RS and Macnaughton J (1999) Should medical students read Plato? *Medical Journal of Australia.* **170**: 125–7.

CHAPTER 6

Training transformed

George Taylor

This chapter describes the development of vocational training for general practice and highlights the potential changes in the future.

Vocational training for general practice, initiated in the mid-1960s, replaced a system of training based on learning by doing under minimal supervision. With vocational training came regulation and conformity and a drive to higher standards.

How training started

Although some schemes were in existence for GP training in the 1950s (for example, the Inverness scheme), most structured programmes of training developed in the late 1960s and early 1970s can be seen very much as a success story for general practice. Their task was clarified in 1972 by the publication of the *The Future General Practitioner*[1] by the Royal College of General Practitioners (RCGP) which defined the role of general practice and outlined those areas that needed to form the curriculum for general practice training.

In 1965 the RCGP had made the case for special training for general practice,[2] a view reiterated in its evidence to the Royal Commission on Medical Education in 1966.[3] In recommending five years of such training, two years were to be spent in general practice. The outcome, however, was the three-year pattern, with only one year being spent in a training practice. In addition, general practice found itself different from all other specialities in two distinct ways. The first was that the requirements for becoming a GP were laid down in statute in the National Health Service (Vocational Training) Regulations 1979,[4] something that does not apply to any other medical speciality. The second was that, unlike other specialities where the relevant royal college defines standards, the RCGP can propose standards but ultimately the body known as the Joint Committee on Postgraduate Training in General Practice (JCPTGP) has overall responsibility as the certifying authority. This committee has representation from the RCGP, the General Medical Services Committee (GMSC) of the BMA and other bodies related to general practice education.

How training is structured

The JCPTGP was formed in 1976 as an independent body that sets the standards for general practice training and issues certificates of 'prescribed' and 'equivalent' experience to doctors who satisfactorily complete periods of training. It is the 'competent authority' for the purposes of the European Union (EU).[5] The Joint Committee, as certifying body, promulgates standards for training at a national level and these are implemented by the universities with medical schools. General practice education committees or their equivalents oversee vocational training in their deanery (the area served by the medical school). Each deanery is required to achieve JCPTGP training standards. In the majority of deaneries two parallel systems of training are in existence. All deaneries have formal training schemes, appointing trainees (in recent years known as registrars) to structured three-year programmes. These schemes, as well as providing a rotation of posts to fulfil the regulations, provide an educational programme geared to general practice.

Alongside this model runs a parallel system where junior doctors organise their own hospital training and then apply for appointment to a trainee year. In the early years of vocational training this risked variation in standards, as trainers could appoint trainees to meet the service needs of their practice rather than on the basis of the quality of the applicants. In more recent years a system by which all applicants are selected at Deanery level against national criteria has been implemented. One deanery, Northern England, has had an agreement with its trainers from the inception of training that trainees, whatever the length of training required, would be appointed through vocational training scheme appointment committees.

Certification

Since 1981, doctors wishing to become GP principals require formal certification.[6] Equally, from 1994 onwards, doctors wishing to act as locums or assistants have had to be certified as having been vocationally trained.[6] Certification should be a straightforward matter for doctors completing a structured three-year scheme. They will have had what is known as 'prescribed' experience, which is training undertaken in the UK in posts recognised for general practice training by an education committee for general practice. Such posts include general medicine, geriatric medicine, medical paediatrics, psychiatry, accident and emergency, general surgery, obstetrics and gynae-cology. They will have had one year in general practice. All such experience must be completed within seven years of the application for certification.

Where doctors have completed training more than seven years previously or held hospital posts not recognised by the education committee for general practice, a certificate of 'equivalent' experience is required. Such doctors may need to submit evidence relating to the service and education provided by their past experience and are required to complete a year in two posts from the list of major specialities noted above. Experience gained in the EU would be recognised for training in the country involved.[6]

Part-time training is an option but one that has been modified by EU regulations.[6] Part-time training must now be equivalent to 60% of full-time training, though this does include the educational programme.

Summative assessment

The need for regular, structured, formative, educational assessment of trainees had been recognised for some years and formed one of the areas of both regional and national assessment of trainers.[7]

To prevent incompetent doctors from being certified, a national assessment standard was introduced in 1996 by the Joint Committee. All trainees must pass a test of knowledge (multichoice question paper), provide a piece of written work (at present an audit), have consulting ability assessed either on video or in a simulated surgery and produce a satisfactory trainer's report (a structured document covering their knowledge, skills and attitudes when in their training practice).

The Membership of the RCGP (MRCGP) examination has been proposed as the voluntary assessment of achievement for trainees in many regions for some years. At present, over 85% of trainees take the MRCGP, despite having to pay an examination fee. A single route by which the MRCGP replaces all sections of summative assessment other than the trainer's report is now available.

Trainers

The need to develop educational skills for general practice trainers has been recognised. Deaneries initially provided courses which covered basic educational theory, teaching and assessment skills. These courses soon became mandatory for all intending trainers, while advanced courses were developed for more experienced trainers. It is now increasingly common for an assessment of teaching skills to be undertaken both prior to first appointment and subsequently. Valid and reliable instruments are being developed to enable this to be achieved in a fair and scientific manner.[8] Trainers themselves formed trainer groups at a local level to provide support and educational help to each other.

Training practices

The training of trainers has gone hand in hand with the need to develop their practices as teaching organisations. Systematic visiting, with a view to accreditation and reaccreditation of such practices, has been in place for over 30 years. Such visits can be used by practices to measure their achievements and to set their standards for future attainment. Many deaneries have expanded these visits to involve, for example, practice managers in their visiting teams. Early visits were very much concerned with practice structure. Reports[9] in the 1970s centred on the physical structure of training practices and on ensuring the provision of what would now be seen as very basic equipment, for example vaginal specula. Good buildings, adequate room for consulting and relevant libraries are now assured. The priorities have moved on to the process of the training itself. This can no longer be something carried out in odd minutes over lunch by the enthusiastic yet unskilled doctor. There should be protected time for teaching when the normal day-to-day tasks of general practice are not allowed to intrude. The curriculum can no longer be the trainer's 20 favourite clinical topics but a programme based on a structured assessment of trainee need. The primary care team, so often a figment of the imagination in the early years, is now drawn into the teaching process. Trainees expect to spend time with team members other than doctors and be educated by and with them.

Course organisers

One of the interesting developments within vocational training has been the evolution of the role of the course organiser. In the early days, they looked after the running of their local scheme and organised the half-day release programme. The half-day release course was initiated for a number of reasons: first to give trainees a central locus for their activities; second to maintain a contact with general practice when they were in their hospital posts; and third to ensure that structured and relevant education was taking place in the early years of vocational training when trainer enthusiasm was sometimes greater than teaching skill. For some time, the role of course organiser tended to be transient: a job taken up by trainers because it was their turn and then handed on to their neighbour. In recent years, course organisers have become more professional, not least because they have developed specialised educational skills in teaching methods, small group leadership, mentoring and management. This expertise is increasingly being recognised, even to the extent of receiving requests from hospitals for them to give structured education to their junior staff.

Course organisers encourage the teaching of consultation skills in general practice.[10] Direct observation, audio-taping and video-taping help both trainer and trainee reflect on what happens during a consultation. Work by Pendleton,[11] Neighbour,[12] Cox[13] and Fraser[14] has illuminated both our understanding of the consultation and how to teach it.

Future developments

The need for flexibility

Vocational training schemes (VTSs) must learn to change with the times. Indeed, schemes perceived to be of a poorer standard or those in less attractive geographical settings risk closure through lack of applicants. Many have examined their organisation to see if it can be made more accessible. Vocational training educational programmes should reflect the needs of modern practitioners. In a time of major change, where practice contracts may replace personal ones and where new models of working using nurse practitioners are developing, there is the clear recognition that the one year spent in practice during training is not enough. In addition, training seeks to provide core skills which doctors can use throughout their professional lives. As many recently trained doctors plan to work less than full time in general practice and may not wish to take on the management role involved in being a partner, different styles of career will develop. The increasing female intake into both medical school and vocational training will demand proper maternity leave arrangements, part-time training options and increased flexibility in the job market.

Although the need to retrain after a break from practice has long been recognised, the facility to do so has been little used. Funds are available for retraining after a prolonged absence from work for doctors who are already certified, but little has been offered in the way of educational support.

There is an increasing recognition of the need for continued education after vocational training.[15] Although there will always be a place for personal development – a course undertaken out of interest rather than need – there is now an understanding that the needs of the practice should drive doctors' continuing education. GP tutors increasingly see their role as developing both personal and practice educational plans. Management skills and research methodology are just two of the areas where increasing numbers of young doctors are undertaking training.

Research

General practice has previously been seen as a backwater for research. The increasing number of GPs wishing to spend some time undertaking research, the recognition of the immense field available for research in primary care and the movement towards primary care in the health service have all brought about a need for the development of research skills in general practice. Some vocational training schemes have developed research posts within their programmes.[16] Others will no doubt wish to follow the lead. The evolution of primary care research networks, research practices (initially funded by the RCGP and now by the NHS) and research fellowships attached to university departments has allowed increasing numbers of GPs to develop a taste and aptitude for research. The next decade will offer more opportunities for general practitioners as this trend continues.

Conclusion

Exposure to general practice increasingly takes place in the undergraduate medical course. There is therefore now an educational continuum which begins early in medical school and goes on until the end of the vocational training scheme. The greater complexity of general practice means that schemes no longer expect to produce the complete GP. Rather, the aim is to equip doctors with the skills of lifelong learning and of coping in an ever-changing world.[17] Vocational training is rising to this challenge.

Changing training for changing times

Introduction

Vocational training for general practice has been in existence for over 30 years. Although great strides have been taken in developing the educational expertise of those involved in its provision over this time, with many having gained formal educational qualifications, the basic structure of training remained remarkably unchanged until March 2000. At this point the funding for training was moved from the general medical services budget into MADEL (the Medical And Dental Educational Levy). It thus came under the direct control of the directors of postgraduate general practice education.[18]

This has allowed major developments to take place. The pragmatic mix of two years as an SHO along with a year in a training practice, which was recognised as a compromise at the outset,[19] can now be modified to include a number of innovations. Posts based in general practice, but allowing secondment to specific hospital departments, hospices and health authority departments of public health, are all now possible. Posts linked to the increasing number of academic departments of general practice can provide research training alongside general practice experience.

More and more it is respectable to admit to wishing to carry out some research or develop new skills to increase your fulfilment and usefulness in practice and to the greater NHS. Higher qualifications can be achieved in extended periods of training, or skills improved by more practical experience either in general practice or in a local hospital. This may well be the route to becoming one of the 'specialised GPs' mentioned in the NHS Plan.[20]

Those doctors who require longer periods of training because of identified educational needs can be more easily accommodated. Returning to general practice after periods either not working or working in another branch of medicine can be eased by provision of supervised retraining.

Flexible training, less than full-time training taken up usually because of domestic commitments, has always been an option in general practice training. It is more easily available now that the funding is held by the directors. This will be of greater importance in the future because of the increasing number of medical students who are now female, some of whom may wish to train flexibly.

GP registrars

GP registrars have changed. They now comprise a small number of doctors who are planning to be principals at once, and some who may do so in a few years. Many of the present generation of doctors, however, do not plan ever to be a principal; their future is as an assistant, a salaried doctor employed by a trust or a primary care group, a retainer scheme doctor or a long-term locum.[21] Many want to do other things alongside general practice and are looking for part-time employment after training that allows this.[22]

Training and its weaknesses

In the past a percentage of trainers employed their registrars directly rather than through a training scheme. Sometimes these doctors were disadvantaged, for example by their weak links with the local vocational training scheme. Since March 2000 all appointments have been centralised to deanery or sub-deanery level. Candidates are appointed using common national criteria and a person specification broadly similar in all parts of the UK.[18] Doctors are still able, however, to undertake their own hospital training programme if they wish (self-construct registrars). In the past this has meant that some inappropriate posts, or posts poor in educational terms, have been used for general practice training. Hospital training has always been recognised as a major weakness in vocational training.[23] The Joint Committee (JCPTGP), the body charged with ensuring the standards of training in the UK, is now taking an increasing interest in this area and how schemes select and evaluate their posts.[24] Because of this we can expect posts that are used for GP training to provide vastly improved education in the next decade. SHOs, for so long the lost tribe in hospital training, are planned to have a system of appraisal introduced into their educational programmes. This mirrors the Record of In-Training Assessment (RITA) process for specialist registrars.[25]

The training practice

What is required in the training practice? Only core skills can be taught and learnt in one short period of training. The first task that is increasingly recognised is that vocational training is only the beginning of learning about general practice, not the end – despite summative assessment! Amongst the skills needing to be developed a vital one is the recognition of the need for lifelong learning, and the development of reflective practice as a norm.

General practice continues to change yet always seems to rise to new challenges. The only way to cope with the never-ending change in the health service is to understand how and why it comes about and how to manage it for your benefit. New GPs need to develop skills in managing themselves and others to be able to function within the NHS. This development should be helped by personal and practice development planning as a tool for continuing professional development.[26] Revalidation with the requirement to collect a portfolio of educational experience[27] and clinical governance[28] should both also facilitate the development of reflective practice.

Consumerism, with the need for professionals to develop a new relationship with society,[29] must be recognised during training and young doctors helped to develop the attributes of the modern professional.[30,31]

After the VTS

General practice training is changing and will have to change more in the future. The recent changes in funding have allowed it to throw off its rigid straitjacket and innovative developments are taking place both in its content and duration. Limited funding for further higher training after the basic three-year cycle has now been found. Whether doctors are taking on posts as young principals or as salaried doctors they have only had a small exposure to the professional life of a general practitioner. They still have a significant need to develop both their professional knowledge base and confidence as practitioners.[32] Higher training will facilitate this. Some young doctors are using this opportunity to develop skills so that they can become 'GPs with a special interest'.

Conclusion

Nothing is more certain than that change will continue to occur. The changes recently taking place in vocational training will go some way in helping young doctors prepare for their professional lives. Further development is still required, however, in the provision of support and development of higher professional education in the early years after training.

Summary

- Vocational training for general practice is highly structured and regulated.
- The present three-year programme is a compromise.
- The original recommendation was for a five-year programme including two years in general practice.
- Recent developments have allowed innovative posts to be developed based in general practice.

References

1   Royal College of General Practitioners (1972) *The Future General Practitioner.* BMA, London.
2   Royal College of General Practitioners (1965) *Special Vocational Training for General Practice: Report from General Practice 1.* RCGP, London.
3   Royal College of General Practitioners (1966) *Evidence to the Royal Commission on Medical Education: Report from General Practice 5.* RCGP, London.
4   National Health Service (Vocational Training) Regulations (1979) Stat Inst 1644. HMSO, London.
5   Official Journal of the European Communities (1993) Volume 36. Council Directive 93/16/EEC.
6   Joint Committee on Postgraduate Education for General Practice (1996) *A Guide to Certification.* JCPTGP, London.
7   Joint Committee on Postgraduate Training for General Practice (1993) *Report of a Working Party on Assessment.* JCPTGP, London.
8   Duggan S, Cox J and O'Halloran C (1998) Formative evaluation of one to one teaching in general practice: development of an instrument. Postgraduate Institute for Medicine and Dentistry, University of Newcastle.
9   Royal College of General Practitioners (1992) *Teaching Practices: Report from General Practice 15.* RCGP, London.
10 Spence J (1960) *The Purpose and Practice of Medicine.* Oxford University Press, Oxford.
11 Pendleton D, Schofield T, Tate P *et al.* (1984) *The Consultation: an approach to learning and teaching.* Oxford University Press, Oxford.
12 Neighbour R (1987) *The Inner Consultation.* MTP Press, Lancaster.
13 Cox J (1993) *An Instrument for Assessment of Videotapes of General Practitioners' Performance* (MD thesis). University of Newcastle upon Tyne.
14 Fraser R (1992) *Clinical Method.* Butterworth-Heinemann, Oxford.
15 Royal College of General Practitioners (1990) *An Educational Strategy for General Practice for the 1990s.* RCGP, London.
16 Education Committee for General Practice (1997) *Annual Report of the Northumbria Vocational Training Scheme for General Practice.* ECGP, University of Newcastle Upon Tyne.

17 Royal College of General Practitioners (1993) *Portfolio Based Learning.* RCGP, London.

18 Field S (2000) Vocational training for general practice. *BMJ Classified.* **19 August.**

19 RCGP (1996) *Evidence to the Royal Commission on Medical Education.* RCGP, London.

20 HMSO (2000) *The NHS Plan.* The Stationery Office, London.

21 Taylor G (2000) Career plans of a cohort of registrars in the Northern Deanery. *Education for General Practice.* **11**(3): 339.

22 Harrison J and van Zwanenberg T (eds) (1998) *GP Tomorrow.* Radcliffe Medical Press, Oxford.

23 RCGP (1993) *The Quality of Hospital Based Education for General Practice.* RCGP, London.

24 JCPTGP (1998) *Recommendations on the Selection and Re-selection of Hospital Posts for General Practice Training.* JCPTGP, London.

25 Conference of Postgraduate Deans (2000) *The SHO Record of Training.* COPMED, London.

26 The Chief Medical Officer (1998) *A Review of Continuing Professional Development in General Practice.* Department of Health, London.

27 RCGP and GPO (2000) *Revalidation for Clinical General Practice.* RCGP, London.

28 Taylor GB (2000) *Has the Introduction of Clinical Governance Facilitated the Development of Quality in General Practice?* School of Education, University of Newcastle, Newcastle upon Tyne.

29 Coulter A (1999) Paternalism or partnership? *BMJ.* **319**: 719–20.

30 Taylor G (2000) What factors will facilitate the development of clinical governance in general practice? Results of a qualitative study. *Journal of Clinical Governance.* **8**(4): 181–5.

31 Irvine D (1999) The performance of doctors: the new professionalism. *Lancet.* **353**: 1174–77.

32 Eraut M (1994) *Developing Professional Knowledge and Competence.* The Farmer Press, London.

PART 2

Preparing the way

CHAPTER 7

Career Start in County Durham

Jamie Harrison and Linda Redpath

Change is inevitable. In a progressive country change is constant.
Disraeli

This chapter describes initiatives in County Durham aimed at understanding and responding to perceived problems in general practice,
including recruitment, stress, and career support and development for
both younger doctors and practice managers.

The local context

Problems in GP recruitment

Over recent years, the distribution of general practitioners has been
relatively even across the UK as a result of the work of the Medical Practices
Committee (MPC). Patients have assumed that, when needed, a general
practitioner would be available.

It therefore shocked one small community near Durham in 1994 when its
general practitioner provision was temporarily withdrawn. A large practice
nearby had medical manpower problems and was unable to continue to
offer personal medical services to the village. Consternation ensued,
questions were asked in Parliament and a solution was found through the
reallocation of the patient list.

This experience coincided with the following.

- Recruitment to vocational training schemes (VTSs) across the Northern Region was down, reflecting national trends.
- Applications to partnership vacancies were low;[1] although retention of general practitioners within County Durham had historically been good, concerns about recruiting the future GP workforce seemed very real.
- More women were in the GP system (with their particular career needs).
- Local co-ops had yet to grasp the out-of-hours issue.
- Many doctors were looking for more flexible contracts of work.

Questions in need of an answer

Concerns about recruitment coincided with wider questioning within the health authority and the local medical committee. Did we know why general practitioners were entering or leaving the country? What part was stress playing in recruiting and retaining doctors? How might better practice management and improved personal career support influence the willingness of younger doctors to put down roots in Durham? How might a culture of better communication and co-operation be developed?

In an attempt to answer these questions, a number of initiatives were put in place. Two were surveys to gain information – on why general practitioners moved practices (joiner–leaver survey) and on how stressed general practitioners felt and why (stress survey). Two were aimed at supporting the early career development of general practitioners (GP Career Start) and practice managers (Manager Career Start). The fifth sought to enhance the effectiveness of existing practice managers (Practice Manager Links).

Joiner–leaver survey

This survey initially took place during the 18 months between 30 June 1994 and 1 January 1996. It was repeated again in 1999. Questionnaires were sent to each group of medical list leavers and joiners, seeking information in five broad areas:

- characteristics of previous practice
- characteristics of current practice
- factors contributing to moving to the present practice
- views on how to attract medical students into general practice
- positive and negative aspects of being a general practitioner.

As the questionnaires contained information which might be deemed sensitive, responders were assured that data would be seen by the health authority in aggregated form only.

What was striking for all four cohorts of joiners and leavers from the studies was how similar their views were on the perfect practice partnership. The right partners, good teamworking and an enhanced quality of life (which also featured as the appropriate location of the practice for them) were consistently seen as being the most important features in choosing a general practice. Conversely, being a training practice, whether or not the area was deprived, and having pleasant premises were regarded as the least important of the practice characteristics offered (Box 7.1).

Box 7.1 Importance of features for choosing a general practice partnership[2] (ranked in descending order of importance)

Partners	1
Good teamwork	2
Quality of life	3
Location	4
Limited out-of-hours	5
Money	6
Local facilities	8
Health authority links	9
Practice IT	10
Low deprivation level	11
Training practice	12

When asked why they had left their previous practice, retirement and changing practices within the Durham area were common responses. The main reasons cited by those joining the list were: to seek financial parity within the partnership, as a result of a practice split and to move to a different location. Respondents appreciated the continuity of care that general practice offered, the personal autonomy (self-employment status) and the generalist role, though it was revealed that the personal freedom a general practitioner had once enjoyed was perceived as being eroded (leavers). In both groups, the respondents valued the teamwork aspect of general practice.

Negative aspects of general practice were perceived by all as excessive patient demand and workload. There was also concern about out-of-hours work, although this was less so for the later cohorts. When asked about attracting general practitioners to County Durham, the general consensus was that the out-of-hours situation would continue to improve and this would have a positive impact on GP recruitment, as would an increase in flexible working arrangements, which was beginning to happen.

In terms of marketing general practice, it was felt that medical students spent too little time with general practitioners to be able to make an informed career choice. More exposure during medical school would improve recruitment, especially where the positive side of general practice was presented.

Stress survey

Increased stress levels have been cited as a major contributor to the fall in the number of those seeking a career in general practice. In particular, many have blamed the 1990 GP contract for the extra stress experienced and consequent low morale,[3] a view supported by Chambers and Belcher[4] and Hannay et al.[5]

A joint medical audit advisory group (MAAG)–local medical committee survey[6] was carried out in October 1995 in order to identify the most common causes of stress for general practitioners in County Durham. The survey was anonymous and achieved a 63% response rate. The top ten causes of stress were found to be:

- emergency calls during surgery hours (74%)
- night calls (65%)
- time pressure (62%)
- working after a sleepless night (58.5%)
- dealing with problem patients (45%)
- worrying about patients' complaints (43%)
- interruption of family life by telephone (42.5%)
- unrealistically high expectations by others (41.5%)
- 24-hour responsibility for patients' lives (37%)
- dividing time between spouses and patients (28%).

These findings were remarkably similar to those reported in stress surveys carried out by Shropshire and Suffolk MAAGs in 1994. They highlight the disruption caused by simultaneous multiple demands made on general practitioners, not least by urgent visit requests occurring during a surgery session. Out-of-hours calls, with the associated disruption of sleep and disturbance to family life, also figure as significant stressors.

Specific comments were made about the difficulty in recruiting GP partners and in acquiring locum support. Some respondents stated that help with finding new partners would be a positive way of increasing morale, as would improving the consequences of out-of-hours working, for example by giving time off following an evening on call, with locum cover for nights and weekends.

In this survey, a pay rise was frequently mentioned as a way of improving morale (offered by 49 of the 196 doctors surveyed). This contrasts with the joiners–leavers survey, where pay was not seen as such a key factor. It should be noted that the two surveys were carried out one year apart.

GP Career Start

Setting the scene

In September 1996, County Durham Health Authority established the two-year, salaried GP Career Start scheme. This aimed to:

- give vocationally trained practitioners the opportunity of a positive and gradual introduction to general practice as a career through continuing education and hands-on experience
- create an appreciation in such general practitioners of the advantages of group practice
- produce a pool of high quality GP manpower within County Durham to succeed to practice vacancies
- provide a further level of training to enable GP Career Start doctors to make the increasingly difficult transition between trainee (registrar) and principal and to acquire further professional qualifications and training.

The full-time salary was set at 80% of net intended GP principal income, with Postgraduate Education Allowance (PGEA) accreditation and pension rights protected. There would be a bonus ('dowry') of 10% of final salary payable should doctors eventually leave GP Career Start to join the County Durham medical list. The scheme was to be doctor-centred in its aims. Unlike those schemes which also looked to help stressed practices or to introduce practice innovation, GP Career Start would concern itself primarily with the personal and professional development of its doctors.

Initially the scheme had expected to employ doctors on a three-year salaried contract, mirroring the VTS scheme. On reflection this seemed too long and risked diverting some from joining partnerships (the opposite of what was intended). A further theoretical point related to the original intention of the pioneers of vocational training who, back in the mid-1960s, had envisaged a five-year period of training for general practice post-registration.[7] Hence, a two-year salaried option post-vocational training was agreed. The first year would be spent in a mentor practice, gaining general experience. The second year would involve more varied locum experience in practices, with protected time to do further training and education, including the option of secondment to the health authority (Box 7.2).

Box 7.2 GP Career Start – two-year scheme

Year 1	*Year 2*
Sessions in one (later two) mentor practice(s)*	50% general practice locums in County Durham
+	+
Half-day release for group education	50% professional and personal development

* The number of half-day sessions can be any number from four to eight depending on contract.

Getting started

Inevitably, new schemes are met with justifiable suspicion. Young general practitioners need to be convinced that such initiatives are viable, can live up to expectations, will meet their particular needs, but will not exploit them.

The mentor practices might fear getting a problem doctor who would be nothing but trouble (on the mistaken assumption that all good doctors went straight into partnerships). They would be asked to pay towards the doctor's salary (around 20%); would it be money well spent?

Seven vocationally trained doctors were recruited to the scheme by interview in June 1996. They were able to choose their mentor practice from a list of 12. Each practice nominated one of its partners to act as the Career Start doctor in the practice to provide ongoing support over the year. Doctors on the Retainer Scheme, who were then only allowed to work for two sessions per week, were encouraged to apply. In the event, two were appointed to work five sessions per week on GP Career Start. In addition, the advert for the scheme in the *British Medical Journal* caught the eye of one general practitioner returning from four years in Budapest:

> I returned to England and had to consider my (career) options again. I knew I wanted to leave London, but otherwise the possibilities were similar to before (assistant, locum, hospital job,

career outside medicine). Partnership would have been a foolish option at this time, particularly in a new area. I started looking in the jobs section of the *BMJ*. How could I not apply!? I asked myself whether this job advertisement was written specially with me in mind![8]

Key issues which the advert touched upon were flexibility, choice and variety.

- Part-time or full-time contracts were offered.
- A choice of mentor practices was available.
- A wide variety of educational options (including electives) were possible.

The first cohort was made up of five women and two men. Contracts were for four or eight practice sessions, with one weekly group session in addition. This cohort contained three types of general practitioner:

- those who had recently left vocational training were cautious about partnerships and conscious of needing more space for education and personal development
- those who had done other things, including locum work and working abroad, but still wanted the option of protected higher professional training
- those on the Retainer Scheme, finding its minimal, two-session per week format failed to equip them for partnership or its equivalent.

The scheme in action

Choice of practices meant exactly that and fortunately no clash of choices occurred in the first year (although it would for later cohorts, where compromises would be needed). Initially, the thought had been to enlist training practices only, but that would have been too restrictive, both in terms of geographical spread and type of practice on offer. In the spirit of flexibility and a learner-centred approach, the doctor would make the choice of mentor practice and live with the consequences.

In the event, on-call duties applied to some practices but not to others – something which should have been made more explicit. Later Career Start doctors would learn to negotiate with their practices, make compromises and do duties in the new out-of-hours co-operatives.

Mentoring worked in markedly different ways in the practices.[9] Those doctors whose mentor was a trainer (in the VTS) had a head start. Non-training practices risked misunderstanding the level of competence of the Career Start doctor, being initially over-protective and too watchful. Formal training in mentoring in the first year was both too little and too late. Developing the mentoring role had been forgotten in the desire to encourage the weekly Career Start doctors' group, something that was picked up by one of its number:

> There is a consensus, certainly within our group, that there is definitely a need for mentors and mentoring. It has also become clear that there is uncertainty about it, and that this is very individual in its nature. Most of us would like personal support and development, professional support and development, and an educational challenge. It is important that the mentoring is focused; we are not just talking about a cosy chat. Hopefully most of us have managed to set up support networks for that. Although (originally) we possibly saw mentors as a crutch to be used in time of crisis only, I, for one, would now perceive it as a way forward for planning my career and a mechanism to help adaptation to change.[8]

The weekly group meeting provided the Career Start doctors with a forum in which to discuss how a future career might be supported and developed. This meeting also provided social, professional and personal support. Clinical cases (and practices) could be discussed and, confidentially, issues raised, and visits made to quiz hospital consultants and non-medical colleagues. The group set its own goals and chose how best to deliver its educational agenda.

The second year of the scheme (year 2) provided a mix of locum-type work, educational attachments and experience of the health authority. Study for MSc or Diploma in Therapeutics options alternated with working in single-handed practices. Attachments to outpatient departments in dermatology, palliative medicine and rheumatology were balanced by an increased exposure to partnerships of differing sizes and to computer systems of varying degrees of complexity.

Since the original 1996 group of seven doctors, five further cohorts of Career Start doctors have been recruited. One major change has been to appoint one doctor per PCG (there are six PCGs in the county), where they work in two nominated practices for two days per week. This corrected a situation where PCGs in the north of the county had a disproportionate number of Career Start doctors. This shift towards greater equity, and more practices involved, sought to pre-empt any feeling that the emerging primary care organisations (PCG/PCTs) were not receiving their fair shares. Equally, the optimum group size has proved to be between six and eight doctors in our experience. It is clear that PCTs might struggle to run a similar scheme if their doctor numbers were much smaller.

Perceived benefits to the members of the Career Start scheme

To date, 19 doctors have left the scheme. Of these, 11 continue in local practice (Box 7.3). It is clear that, even five years after leaving vocational training, the career requirements of general practitioners are both varied and in transition. For some, partnership remains a long-term goal; for others, flexible salaried options are what is required.

Box 7.3 Career paths of 19 Career Start leavers

County Durham
Principal	6
Retainee	3
Salaried post	2

Wider NHS
Principal	3
Retainee	2
Salaried post	2
Locum	1

One Career Start leaver, who is now in a partnership which includes two other ex-Career Start doctors, reflected on her first year of the scheme in the following terms.

Achievements in past year

- Move to new area.
- Stability.
- Increased clinical confidence/work experience/education.
- Support from within mentor practice.
- Support from peer group.
- Look in further detail at the running of a practice.
- Specific skills such as computer literacy.
- Opportunities to explore possibilities for the future.

Both past and present Career Start doctors found the idea of becoming a partner immediately on leaving their VTS daunting.[10,11] For them, Career Start offered space and time for personal and professional development. By the end of the scheme they felt prepared for partnership, and able to meet its challenges and responsibilities. However, what influenced their next career choice was a mix of three factors – the range of career options, the need to balance home and work life, and the size of commitment that partnership entails. These factors are therefore not about feelings of confidence, but rather about whether, given that a choice exists, partnership best fits the doctor's circumstances.

Manager Career Start and Practice Manager Links

In recognition of the need to support general practice and general practitioners through better practice management, two schemes were devised.

Manager Career Start was modelled on the GP Career Start scheme. The two-year Manager Career Start scheme began in April 1997 with the aims of providing structured and comprehensive training for individuals; providing a resource to individual practices; and shaping the future development of practice management in the county. Three trainees and three mentor practice managers were recruited to the scheme, and the trainees received both practical and educational support. All three trainees are now working in a managerial capacity in primary care. Two are fully established practice managers (one working in County Durham and one in a neighbouring health authority area), and the third is clinical governance manager for one of the local primary care groups, working with a range of different practices. The demise of GP fundholding and the resultant practice management redundancies meant that the scheme was not extended beyond the first cohort of trainees.

Practice Manager Links was also launched in 1997 following the successful implementation of a scheme linking up practice nurses in the county. Practice managers were recruited to the six localities and spent approximately 12 hours per month supporting managers new to the role. They also provided a conduit for two-way communication between practices, and between practices and the health authority, and they helped in sharing good practice and in assessing staff training needs. The Practice Manager Links function continues in the six localities (now PCGs), and the establishment of the role has been helpful in raising the profile of practice management in the county. When PCGs were set up their board structure did not provide for formal input from practice managers. Practice Manager Links was seen by most of the PCGs as a useful mechanism for engaging practice managers in the work of the PCG and bringing a practice management perspective to numerous issues.

Summary

- Problems in GP morale and recruitment appeared in the mid-1990s.
- County Durham Health Authority instigated a range of initiatives.
- The joiners–leavers survey found reasons why doctors left and joined practices.
- The stress survey explored issues of morale and wellbeing.
- GP Career Start is a two-year salaried scheme for non-principals.
- Manager Career Start was a similar scheme to train practice managers.
- A fixed-term salaried post with training and support is attractive to many.

References

1   Medical Practices Committee (1995) *Medical Practices Committee Recruitment Survey.* MPC, London.
2   Redpath L and Harrison J (2000) GP principal recruitment and retention in County Durham: a comparison of joiner–leaver surveys from 1996 and 1999. *Education for General Practice* **11**: 391–6.
3   Sutherland VJ and Cooper CL (1992) Job stress, satisfaction, and mental health among general practitioners before and after introduction of the new contract. *BMJ.* **304**: 1545–8.
4   Chambers R and Belcher J (1993) Work patterns of general practitioners before and after the introduction of the 1990 contract. *British Journal of General Practice.* **43**: 410–12.
5   Hannay D, Usherwood T and Platts M (1992) Workload of general practitioners before and after the new contract. *BMJ.* **304**: 614–18.
6   Durham Primary Care Resource Unit/Durham LMC (1995) *County Durham GP Stress Survey.* MAAG, Durham.
7   Royal Commission on Medical Education (1968) *Todd Report.* HMSO, London.
8   Johnston T (1998) speaking at the GP Tomorrow Conference, Royal County Hotel, Durham, 3 October.
9   Bregazzi R, Harrison J and van Zwanenberg T (2000) Mentoring new GPs: experience from GP Career Start in County Durham. *Education for General Practice.* **11**: 58–64.
10 Bonsor R, Gibbs T and Woodward R (1998) Vocational training and beyond – listening to voices from a void. *British Journal of General Practice.* **48**: 915–18.
11 Bregazzi R and Harrison J (2002) Committing to partnership: experience from GP Career Start in County Durham. *Education for Primary Care.* **13**: 42–7.

CHAPTER 8

The South London VTA scheme seven years on

Lesley Delacourt and Richard Savage

> This chapter describes the Vocationally Trained Associate scheme and its impact after seven years.

Introduction

The Vocationally Trained Associate (VTA) scheme was set up by the South London Organisation of Vocational Training Schemes (SLOVTS) in Lambeth, Southwark and Lewisham (LSL), South London in 1994, making it one of the oldest and most established salaried schemes in the country. The scheme's explicit aims are:

- to attract newly qualified doctors to South London by giving them positive experiences of inner-city general practice
- to address the need of doctors leaving vocational training schemes (VTSs) for a fourth year of training in general practice
- to help stressed inner-city practices at times of change or development.

Since the scheme began in 1994:

- exactly 50 GPs have been in the scheme
- of these, 20 are still working as GP principals and two as salaried (PMS) doctors in LSL
- a further seven are still working in LSL as assistants or locums
- VTAs have contributed approximately 120 person-years to general practice in LSL over the last seven years
- over half of all LSL practices have now had a VTA

- ex-VTAs are now senior partners in LSL, VTS course organisers, GP tutors, mentors to other GPs or training to become trainers.

The VTA scheme demonstrates that young GPs, given sufficient support in the years immediately after vocational training, can be successfully recruited and retained into stressful inner-city practices.

The VTA scheme's working week is as follows:

- seven sessions working in two busy inner-city practices
- one session in a facilitated peer group meeting
- one session for individual project, research or audit for presentation to the rest of the group
- one session for individual personal or professional development.

The following account is a development of articles originally published in *Education for General Practice*.[1-3]

Background

Falling numbers of applicants for VTS nationwide,[4,5] coupled with widespread concern that substantial numbers of medical graduates might be leaving the profession,[6] prompted Guy's and St Thomas' VTS to examine how its registrars perceived their future. The review showed that the majority were unwilling to make an immediate commitment to becoming principals in general practice. Some registrars thought they still lacked the necessary clinical skills. Others felt that the rapid changes occurring in general practice made it a less attractive career choice than they had anticipated. They were apprehensive about the perceived challenges of working in inner-city general practice.[7] They were not ready for managerial responsibilities and they were discouraged by the perceived lack of flexibility in partnership.[8]

A review of the choices of registrars leaving all four South London schemes (set out in a personal communication from the Chair of SLOVTS to the LSL Health Authority) found that many registrars wanted 'time out' to recover from the pressures of years of curricular and examination-driven study before committing themselves to partnerships. Up to 30% of the scheme's registrars went abroad to work as doctors. Others became locums or assistants, which gave them opportunities to practise and sharpen their clinical skills and avoid the managerial, financial and emotional commitments of entering a partnership.

There appeared to be a need for an extra, structured year of professional development in general practice. This would provide exposure to the complex interpersonal, financial and managerial aspects of partnership and to the variety of arrangements for delivering primary healthcare. It would also enable registrars to practise making informed choices about their professional futures. SLOVTS was keen to find a way to enable registrars to develop into confident and well-rounded general practitioners.[9] With collaboration, support and encouragement from LSL Health Authority, SLOVTS established the VTA scheme for GPs as an alternative to an immediate partnership or locum work.

The scheme was initially funded by a London Initiative Zone grant, allocated as part of extra money available to primary care in London, following the Tomlinson Report.[10] Subsequently mainstream funding was allocated by the health authority, supplemented in recent years by contributions from practices. For practices, the contribution required compares favourably with the cost of employing locums. The scheme remains subsidised by the health authority as practices between them contribute approximately one third of the GPs' salaries plus on-costs.

In LSL, the health authority recognised three factors affecting the local recruitment crisis:

- the changing expectations of young GPs
- the lack of a wide range of contractual arrangements available to them
- the high proportion of local GPs approaching retirement and the need to replace them with a cohort of younger doctors.

The VTA scheme is one of several initiatives supported by the health authority to help address the serious projected shortfall of GPs. Other initiatives aim to make it easy for potential GPs to access information on vacancies, to create a sense of welcome and support:

- 'GP Opportunities' – this is a 'one-stop shop', a centralised database of all local GP vacancies for which SLOVTS places corporate advertising and organises recruitment information from practices
- 'New Practitioner Support' – a professional development package for any GP new to the area, which includes induction, an overview of public health in LSL, access to local support networks and New or Young Practitioner groups
- an annual New Practitioners' Conference, held for the last five years and attracting up to 90 participants.

All initiatives are open to any GP working in LSL in any capacity for their first three years.

The structure of the VTA scheme

The VTA scheme aims to help participating practices to cope better by providing the continuity of three or four weekly sessions of extra doctor time as a 'breathing space', to allow practices to develop.

Practices applying for the placement of a VTA need to:

- fulfil certain criteria on staffing levels and services provided, so that VTAs experience practices with basic facilities in place
- have a list size averaging between 1700 and 2800 patients per principal
- have clearly identifiable causes of stress which would be alleviated or at least addressed through the attachment of a VTA.

Applications from practices were initially screened by representatives of the health authority and the local medical committee. In recent years each of LSL's six primary care groups have shortlisted four practices, using the same criteria above.

The scheme aims to encourage young general practitioners to become principals in the inner city and sets out to achieve this by:

- encouraging and supporting the VTAs' professional development through protected time and a peer support group
- providing a positive experience of inner-city practice
- giving them choices of practices to work in
- allowing them to discover the range of practices in South London.

Professional support

Based on the conviction that structured support is a crucial element for the health of a general practitioner, various support systems are built in to the scheme:

- the VTA peer group
- a mentor in one of their two practices
- the co-ordinator of the scheme.

Whatever the problem or concern, someone with the right resources exists within the network to listen and, if appropriate, to give advice to the VTA. This experience encourages VTAs to replicate similar networks around themselves throughout their careers.

The group

The members shape and determine how the group works. Some VTAs prefer a more structured approach with guest speakers and previously agreed topics; others appreciate more unstructured sessions. As attendance at group sessions is an obligatory part of the working week, VTAs cannot 'vote with their feet' if they do not like the way the group is working. Their responsibility is to confront what they dislike and change the way the group works. In order for each person to get maximum value, they need to say what they want, need or dislike. With honesty and goodwill, each of the groups evolves its own way of working which is flexible, tolerant and understanding of the problems any one of its members might be facing at work.

Groups work best when all VTAs in each cohort started together. Recent cohorts have run from October to September in order to take advantage of the time when many young GPs are looking for posts. Starting together and an early 'away day' out of London helps VTA groups to gel. Through this structured start they discover the value of peer support for solving problems, confronting issues, analysing critical incidents, and 'dumping' and coping with stress and anxiety. VTAs gain valuable experience for practice meetings by rotating the responsibility for chairing group meetings.

The mentors

Each VTA has a mentor in one of their two practices. The mentor arranges an induction into the practice and provides regular protected time for the VTA to discuss any clinical, professional or practice issue, or personal issue if their work is affected. The mentoring system works well in most cases. Some VTAs choose experienced practice managers as their mentors. Some mentors are experienced GP trainers, but most are non-trainers. An unexpected benefit has been the interest generated amongst mentors in becoming trainers, as many find it a challenge and appreciate the responsibility of the role. This is particularly encouraging given the local shortage of trainers. Others become mentors on another LSL scheme.

VTAs and mentors used the time creatively and in fact the teaching aspect of training was only a small part of the mentor's role, so much so that many mentors said they gained at least as much as they gave. In some cases mentoring developed into 'co-mentoring' in the later part of the year as trust and confidence grew.

The co-ordinator

The co-ordinator acts as advocate for the VTAs, liaising between the scheme and the practices, between the scheme and the health authority and PCGs, and providing resources as appropriate. The co-ordinator also acts as the group facilitator, ensuring that the group provides an atmosphere conducive to reflection, pooling of experiences and learning. Both the co-ordinators employed over the seven years of the scheme had educational, groupwork and management experience (one had practice management experience). The early decision not to employ a GP was deliberate: VTAs appreciate how much knowledge they possess as a group when they are unable to turn to an experienced GP as the 'expert' facilitating the group.

Choosing practices by negotiating with peers

The VTAs start their year by making choices. Presented with a list of practices (usually four or five more practices than are needed), VTAs make their own personal shortlists of practices using information such as list size, location, practice activities, etc. They then arrange to visit them. Visits enable VTAs to form their own impression of the level of organisation in the practice, the premises, the interests and personalities of GPs and their staff, and what their role in the practice might be.

The group then negotiates who works where. The process highlights the importance of honest, assertive, clear communication and skilful negotiation; a good grounding for being in a partnership. Negotiating with people who (at that stage) are strangers but who eventually become close and supportive colleagues is a powerful beginning for working in the group, a vital component of the VTA year.

Discovering the opportunities available to doctors working in South London

The available practices vary greatly: large or single-handed practices offering a great range of services or wishing to do so; in suburbia or in tower blocks; well organised or struggling. This range allows VTAs to discover and experience different approaches to healthcare and styles of delivery. In this way they are able to formulate their own values and their preferred working arrangements.

VTAs have the opportunity to work in London without having to make long-term commitments at an early stage. Initially, many VTAs are uncertain about the challenging problems of inner-city practice. During the VTA year, they discover the strengths of the local networks for personal support. Access to comprehensive training also provides educational opportunities for continuing personal and professional development. Educational sessions offer a wide variety of presentations by guest speakers or visits to local and national organisations.

Responses from VTAs

VTAs are required to complete progress reports throughout their year. Almost unanimously, they are extremely enthusiastic about the year, with quotes ranging from 'It has been an excellent stepping stone into partnership' to 'The VTA year confirmed I am in the right career and most of the time I feel I am in the right place. Working in the inner city is fascinating and challenging but at times extremely distressing ... I'll be very sad to leave the scheme.'

For those who travel or work overseas after qualifying or who come from hospital jobs or from starting a family, it offers a welcome reintroduction to general practice. VTAs feel their skills are refreshed and they realise what they can offer a practice: 'I feel I have re-established my consulting style, confidence and enjoyment of general practice after four years working overseas ... I feel ready to enter a partnership and look forward to doing so in LSL.'

Some are surprised how much they changed their minds about their 'ideal' practice as the year progressed. Many are acutely aware of the difference between their 'first impressions' of their chosen practices and the subsequent reality; a recurring and always useful learning experience.

The exposure to stressed inner-city practices, balanced with the supportive network, gives VTAs an opportunity to explore and debate how they might avoid 'burnout'. They test the systems and boundaries they would need to put in place in order to keep healthy, while still giving generously to patients and their practices. Often the sources of stress in the practices emanated from leadership, management and financial issues. VTAs therefore become more aware of these issues, start to discover what type of practice feels right for them to work in and identify skills they need to learn to make an effective contribution.

The security of a year's contract with minimal on-call and no responsibility for the running of the practice enabled the VTAs to cope with the highs and lows so common at this stage of their personal lives.

Professionally, they appreciate the continuity of working in the practices which allows them to get to know their patients and to integrate into practice teams.

The VTA experience was summed up by a VTA who said:

> Personally it has been an excellent year that has bridged the gap
> between finishing the VTA and feeling ready to start as a partner,

which I didn't at the beginning. It was good to have a structure
and a supportive group and to be in two practices for the year ...
getting a clearer picture of the kind of practice I want to be part
of.'

Responses from practices

Practices are also asked to report on their experiences at the end of their
VTA year.

All but a minority report that they greatly value the help from an extra
doctor. The dissatisfied practices had not expected the lack of control they
had over the VTA: 'We hoped we were receiving the equivalent of a guaranteed locum for three sessions a week for a year ... and we were not in
control,' or were surprised by the emphasis the scheme gave to personal and
professional development: 'We expected to have a VTA for about 44 weeks
out of the year and we were rather surprised at the amount of time we lost
her due to study leave ...'

Practices note the different approaches to work that VTAs can represent.
Their response can be wryly envious: 'The scheme is very protective of the
VTA's boundaries and perhaps we can learn from that. Perhaps if we were
able to ring-fence our responsibilities we would not feel so overwhelmed,'
suggesting that general practice may need to change to accommodate the
ways that young GPs prefer to work, rather than vice versa.

Practices that clearly define tasks for themselves, such as changes to
premises or computerisation, are most likely to feel that the time freed up by
the VTA is usefully spent. Many other tasks are also successfully completed,
often with the direct involvement of the VTA: clinical governance issues are
addressed, protocols and clinics are developed and established, medical
records are overhauled, management procedures are audited and changed.
Those practices that have less clear plans or projects sometimes found
themselves even more aware of their original level of stress at the end of the
placement since they all too easily absorbed the extra sessions into routine
timetabling. Some decide that after experiencing extra doctor time they
would not want to return to their initial workload and therefore looked for
opportunities to increase their medical staffing. Several practices reported on
general workload, and how the presence of the VTA affected it: 'The help
with the workload has enabled our general mood and behaviour to be less
frenetic,' and the two-way nature of the learning experience was demonstrated: 'We have appreciated the experience of a more recently qualified
doctor in keeping us up to date.'

For some practices, the arrival of a VTA is quite a shock to the system, particularly for the smaller practices where GPs become used to working in isolation. Sharing their patients was a new experience: 'I found it difficult to let go of "my" patients and then ended up being delighted that at times I could offload the "heart-sinks" ... I feel much more at ease with the possibility of having an assistant and think that my mind is somewhat more open clinically.'

In their report to SLOVTS, one practice summarised the experience by saying they:

> ... appreciated the chance to work with a young energetic doctor who practised good medicine, was very willing and who adapted painlessly to our methods and policies. He was able to make positive suggestions and yet understand that what was required was simply to get on with the workload so as to reduce the stress for the other doctors. We were rejuvenated by his freshness and fun!'

Conclusions and the future

The VTA scheme was set up to facilitate the transition from registrar to confident GP. The scheme has meant that 22 newly trained GPs, out of a total of 50 who have been on the scheme, have stayed on as principals, assistants or salaried doctors in South London. The VTAs are enthusiastic about the educational and professional development opportunities available on the scheme as well as the chance to experience the diversity of general practice.

From group discussions and feedback from individual VTAs, it is clear that a young GP's commitment can be expressed in many ways. Not wanting to be a full-time general practitioner, particularly in today's stressful climate, does not signal a lack of commitment; neither does a hesitation to settle into a partnership 'for life'. Many young GPs decide that the pursuit of a further interest is very important to them and want to combine practising as a general practitioner with serious pursuit of other interests (for example in hospital work, research, teaching or training). The 'market' is now responding to the need to provide the kinds of flexible working arrangements which will keep these highly motivated and dedicated young doctors in general practice.

The participating stressed practices gain three or four extra weekly sessions of high quality doctor time and the opportunity to address their problems and are pleased to have the continuity and reliability of help.

Some learn of the different perspectives and professional expectations of young doctors – and how general practice is changing to accommodate them. Many are able to undertake necessary developments in a less stressful way because of the VTA's contribution.

The local PCGs have benefited by increasing the pool of enthusiastic young doctors while the health authority has been able to demonstrate its concern and support for local practitioners under stress. The VTA scheme gives practices the opportunity to learn about themselves.

The VTA scheme's success has been that it has assisted the professional development of young GPs, alleviated some of the stresses felt by host practices and contributed highly qualified doctors to redress some of the health authority's local shortage. The scheme has provided a template which has been replicated in other parts of the country.

The VTA scheme remains popular with twice as many applicants each year as posts. 'Word of mouth' results in several applications each year, with many applicants choosing the scheme because of the positive experiences of their VTA friends and colleagues. However, with the advent of PMS posts, young GPs now have a huge choice of salaried posts, many of which are based on the VTA and other early schemes and the scheme's ability to recruit successfully may not continue.

Opportunities to pool resources for joint recruitment and professional development with the health authority and PCGs are currently being pursued.

Summary

- The scheme demonstrates that the needs of young GPs for time out after exam pressure can be made compatible with the need to recruit and retain doctors to the inner city.
- Support and professional development are essential to achieving this.
- The scheme prepares GPs for practice life by providing opportunities for negotiation, developing chairing and presentation skills and experimenting.

References

1   Salmon E and Savage R (1997) A professional development year in general practice – the VTA scheme. *Education for General Practice*. **8**: 112–20.
2   Salmon E and Savage R (1997) The VTA scheme: outcomes after the first 2 years – the VTAs. *Education for General Practice*. **8**: 191–8.
3   Salmon E and Savage R (1997) The VTA scheme: outcomes after the first 2 years – the impact of practices. *Education for General Practice*. **8**: 199–205.

4   Donald AG (1990) Retreat from general practice. *BMJ*. **301**: 1060.

5   Burrows D and Gould M (1994) Dramatic fall in UK trainees. *Pulse*. **54**: 2–3.

6   Brearley S (1993) How many doctors does Britain need by 2010? *BMJ*. **306**: 155.

7   Lorentzon M, Jarman B and Bajekal M (1994) *Report of the Inner City Task Force of Royal College of General Practitioners*. RCGP, London.

8   Beardow R, Cheung K and Styles WM (1993) Factors influencing the career of general practitioner trainees in North West Thames Regional Health Authority. *British Journal of General Practice*. **43**(376): 449–52.

9   Vaughan C (1995) Career choices for Generation X. *BMJ*. **311**: 525–6.

10   Tomlinson B (1992) *Report of the Inquiry into London's Health Service, Medical Education and Research*. HMSO, London.

CHAPTER 9

Academic training in London

George Freeman, Jon Fuller, Sean Hilton and Frank Smith

... proceed, illustrious Youth,
And Virtue guard thee to the Throne of Truth.
The Scholar's Life

This chapter outlines the context for an academic GP career and describes the London Academic Training Scheme (LATS) for GPs who have completed their three years of vocational training.

Academic general practice

General practice is perhaps the oldest clinical discipline in medicine, but as a distinct academic discipline, it is almost the newest. Academic general practice is contemporary with the NHS itself; in 1998 the proto-academic department at Edinburgh was 50 years old. An important stimulus to development was the formation of the College of General Practitioners in 1952. Whereas the Edinburgh department was headed by the first professor of general practice in the world (appointed in 1963), the establishment of academic departments of general practice in all medical schools in the UK has been quite a slow process. Only in 1996 was a professor finally appointed in one of the oldest universities, Cambridge.

The idea of general practice as an academic discipline has only gradually become accepted even by general practitioners themselves. Not all are members of their own College, unlike other medical disciplines. There has been an atmosphere of suspicion and even mistrust between service GPs and academic GPs who were seen as a disparate body, living in ivory towers.[1] Increasing self-confidence in academic general practice, however, and more opportunities to work together have helped break barriers down. Even so, there is some way to go before an academic arm can be said to be an established part of general practice. One factor in this is the rarity of academic GPs. There is approximately only one for every 50 service colleagues. The comparable figure in hospitals is one academic for every 3.5 service consultants.[2]

Careers in academic general practice

The absence of an established career structure for academic general practitioners applies equally to those who want to work full time in university departments or part time, primarily based in service practice. Other chapters describe initiatives which help bridge the gap between vocational training and service general practice. The gulf in the academic career path is even greater.

While it might be logical for academic departments to recruit their junior grade (lecturers) from service general practice, the consequent drop in salary is unthinkable to most young principals. Lecturers therefore have tended to be appointed just after completion of vocational training. A number of problems face these young doctors. A lecturer's contract is normally for only three years. In this time the lecturer is supposed to:

- master the art of service general practice as a young principal
- become an accomplished teacher able to train and lead others
- learn research skills to the extent of setting up a personal research programme
- write this up in the form of an MD or PhD thesis.

With the increased dependence of universities on research funding, research training is now even more demanding. Some universities expect young academics to have a doctorate before taking up a lectureship. A number of three-year national academic training posts have been made available for competition. They are funded jointly by the Department of Health and the Medical Research Council. GPs with no previous academic training are disadvantaged when applying for such posts.

One large hurdle facing those undertaking research is the absence of a research tradition in general practice. Role models are few and sources of help, even from academic colleagues, are hard to find. This is also the time when young academic GPs are marrying, raising families and establishing households.

Developing a research culture

The prospects for developing a research culture in general practice have improved, with increasing opportunities for a wider range of GPs to undertake research and teaching. A number of practice research networks are becoming established with financial support from the NHS. Nevertheless there is still little research input into vocational training. Although GP registrars are required to complete a project, usually an audit,[3] their trainers are often ill-equipped to guide them.

There is a good argument for all GPs to receive some academic training at the start of their careers, since these are increasingly relevant to clinical governance and to management in primary care groups and trusts. Such academic skills awareness will lead to better recruitment to academic departments and this is important for general practice as a whole. Within medical schools, departments compete for prestige and resources. High standards will enable recognition and funding which will feed back into more support for service practice.

In fact there has been a widespread and growing recognition of the need for academic training for at least a decade.[4] There are notable examples from other countries. The Robert Wood Johnson Fellowship scheme in the USA funds young family practitioners for two or three years in an academic department to develop research and teaching skills. Nearer home, the Royal College of General Practitioners (RCGP) has been able to create a small number of research training fellowships for young principals.

An experimental academic training post started in Southampton in 1992. Although limited to one post, a number of useful lessons were learned:

- the need for separate service and academic mentorship
- the problems of balancing time allocation between service and academic work
- the relevance of the initial academic training was constrained by the lack of clinical experience in general practice.

Opportunities in London

A completely new opportunity arose in London with the London Initiative Zone Educational Incentives Programme (LIZ EI) in 1993.[5] The London Academic Training Scheme (LATS) was conceived in a meeting between two of the authors (George Freeman and Sean Hilton) and the late Bill Styles, then Regional Adviser in General Practice for North West Thames and Chairman of the RCGP Council. LIZ EI offered an unprecedented scale of funding, albeit short-term. Well-worked-out schemes were at a premium. The LATS proposal, with its well-defined objectives and an achievable methodology, was agreed as one of the early initiatives funded by a top slice from the LIZ EI allocation to the various districts. Crucially, London's geographic concentration of academic departments offered training expertise covering a wide range of different research skills.

The scheme was offered to young doctors who had completed their GP vocational training. LATS was a full-time year. It included three clinical sessions each week in general practice to maintain clinical skills and, most importantly, to make sure that the research and teaching was firmly based in service realities. There was also a commitment to improve clinical standards within the LIZ. One way of doing this was to attach LATS academic GP registrars (as they became known) to practices with academic potential, but which were not already designated as training practices.

Aims and objectives

The learning objectives (Box 9.1) showed a dominance of research over teaching and service ones. This does not imply that research is more important than teaching, nor that service needs should be ignored. General practice already has a fine tradition of postgraduate education with well-established methodology. The reverse is true for research, where there is much ground to make up. We have made no apology, therefore, for insisting the majority of LATS is directed at research. This research, nevertheless, must be relevant to service practitioners.

Box 9.1 Learning objectives

LATS should enable the academic GP registrar to:
- overview the research process
- discern soluble and relevant research questions
- undertake a focused literature review
- be aware of both qualitative and quantitative research designs and match these to research questions
- identify common methodological pitfalls including errors of sampling and of measurement, bias and confounding problems
- present a research idea to a peer group and to an expert and then modify the plan
- design, complete and begin to disseminate her/his own research project

- know where to find and how to use expert help
- be experienced in one-to-one and small group teaching both with undergraduates and postgraduates, including multidisciplinary groups
- gain familiarity with inner-city practice and how this can link with an academic department
- make an informed career choice about personal involvement with academic general practice.

Process

With funding for 12 registrars, each of the eight London University departments of general practice was able to participate in the inaugural intake in 1995. There were 32 applicants.

The educational plan was simple. Seven half-day sessions each week were allocated to academic training, of which one would be a group meeting with all LATS registrars. The three remaining sessions were to be spent in general practice.

The half-day group session was led by a different department each term to take advantage of their contrasting skills and expertise. The initial plan was that there would be academic taught sessions on alternate weeks and registrar-led support under the guidance of a mentor in the intervening weeks.

Academic registrars were expected to take part in a departmental project and, if possible, undertake one project of their own under supervision. The scheme was of course new to all the departments and supervisors had to be found. The process for selection varied. Some were volunteers and some were allocated the job!

Funding

The case for funding had to be carefully argued. It was eventually agreed that it would cover:

- the salaries of the registrars
- academic supervision at senior lecturer rates for one session each week from each department
- an additional one session per week of academic supervision for the department running the group session
- a small amount of administrative time.

The registrars themselves were employed by the universities, who provided accommodation. Therefore all the salary costs attracted the university indirect costs surcharge of 40%. Salaries and overheads were by far the largest items in the budget. Smaller sums were set aside to cover the expenses of the visiting teachers, the travel and educational needs of the registrars, and the evaluation. The total budget in the first year for 12 registrars was nearly £600 000. The practices were given virtually free assistants, the registrars being salaried by the medical school. The practices only had to pay £80 per month to defray the cost of medical defence subscription and expenses such as car mileage.

Initial evaluation

One strong point of all LIZ EI schemes was the insistence on properly funded evaluation from the start. There were four domains that needed to be assessed – the registrars themselves, the departments and supervisors, the general practices and the half-day weekly group session. Data were collected at the beginning, middle and end of each year using questionnaires, telephone interviews and special meetings of the group of supervisors.

Twelve registrars were appointed in year 1. Nine stayed for the whole year with three leaving after nine months. Ten of the registrars assessed their practice attachments as very successful. Their practices were correspondingly enthusiastic. Two principals felt that communication had been poor between themselves, their registrars and the host department.

All the registrars undertook at least one research project. Confidence in their skills increased as the year went on. Although they realised they had much to learn, they increasingly became attracted to an academic career. Six months after they had left the scheme, seven were practising in inner London and six of these had a full-time or part-time academic post. One registrar attained an academic post outside London. The initial results were thus very encouraging.

The growth of the scheme

The LATS registrars made a significant contribution to their host departments. Departments were sufficiently encouraged by the scheme to press for an enlargement in the second year and 19 registrars were appointed. In year 2 virtually all departments hosted at least two registrars and a ninth department was added, with the inclusion of the University of Westminster.

At departmental level the increased numbers were welcome as registrars were able to support each other and learn together. The use of an intensive research methods overview allowed the registrars' real learning needs to be determined,[6] and enabled a realistic and relevant educational programme to be devised. The total group size of 20, however, proved rather large for the half-day release sessions. There was good research output, improved experience of teaching and training about teaching, and better relationships with the GP practices. Seventeen of the doctors wished to continue in academic practice in inner London.

In year 3 the scheme returned to a group of 12. This was felt to offer the ideal size for group sessions. The evaluation had suggested that one or two registrars per department was probably more realistic in terms of availability of supervision. Another strong field of applicants allowed 12 more to be appointed.

The end of the three-year LIZ EI programme also meant the end of London-wide funding earmarked for general practice and which bridged the educational and research budgets. However, LATS was able to continue on a smaller scale for two further years with six registrars in each intake, one for each of the academic departments which themselves were reduced in number by amalgamation. Strong competition for the available posts continued, with enquiries from all over the UK. The fifth cohort completed their LATS posts in the autumn of 2000.

Outcomes

The immediate outcomes have been good throughout the five years. LATS registrars have been accepted and welcomed in all the London academic departments of general practice. They have contributed to the research output of these departments and they made a valuable contribution to teaching. They have encouraged departmental links with a new range of inner-city practices. On leaving the scheme the majority have stayed in London and are linked with academic departments.

We contacted the 49 former members of the first four cohorts in 2000 and had full replies from 37. Of these 32 (86%) were working in London and 34 (92%) were in general practice. Nineteen were working five or more service sessions per week. Twenty (54%) were currently members of academic departments. These included 16 with research sessions and 11 who were managing teaching programmes. At least one of the non-respondents has since started a higher academic training fellowship in Canada. A collection of peer-reviewed papers appeared in a special supplement to *Family Practice*.[7] This supplement included the first official evaluation report.

Over a five-year period, LATS-trained academic GPs have either embarked on promising academic careers or are making useful and visible contributions to service practice, often through links with academic departments.

LATS is but one of a number of post-vocational training schemes. It has specific and relatively constrained objectives concerned with academic skills. After the good fortune of generous funding from the LIZ EI, the challenge now is to secure future support from the universities, the NHS or both. There may need to be a greater contribution from the practices. At least one promising 'son of LATS' was reported recently in the *Career Focus* section of the *BMJ Classified*. This is in Warwick and so is styled WATS![8]

For academic departments, LATS is like the answer to a prayer and ideally should be extended across the country. For service general practice, such schemes hold out the possibility of encouraging and supporting evidence-based medicine. For GP registrars LATS has enabled informed choice about academic activity and careers and also about inner-city practice. For general practice as a whole there has been an injection of academic skills which engender self-confidence and the prospect of GPs developing and offering better quality of care to their patients.

Summary

- General practice is only just emerging as an academic discipline.
- Academic GPs have no established career structure.
- There is a significant gulf between leaving vocational training and starting an academic GP career.
- LATS acts as a fourth year of vocational training.
- LATS provides academic mentorship, protected time and training in research skills.
- LATS has been successful in launching young GPs on an academic career.
- Academic general practice injects skills and confidence into service general practice.

References

1   Allen J, Wilson A, Fraser R and Pereira Gray D (1993) The academic base for general practice: the case for change. *BMJ.* **305**: 719–22.

2   Handysides S (1994) A career structure for general practice. *BMJ.* **308**: 253–6.

3   Pereira Gray D, Murray S, Hasler J *et al.* (1997) The summative assessment
     package: an alternative view. *Education for General Practice.* **8**: 8–15.
4   Association of University Departments of General Practice (1993) *A Career
     Structure for Academic General Practice.* AUDGP, Leicester.
5   Department of Health (1993) *Making London Better.* HMSO, London.
6   Pitts J and White P (1994) Learning objectives in general practice: identifica-
     tion of 'wants and needs'. *Education for General Practice.* **5**: 59–65.
7   Freeman G (1998) The London Academic Training Scheme (LATS). *Family
     Practice.* **15**(Suppl. 1): 1–44.
8   Jatsch W, Piercy J, Martin J and Deegan T (2001) A year as academic general
     practioner registrars. *BMJ Classified.* **14 April**: 2–3.

CHAPTER 10

Personal Medical Services (PMS) – their contribution to recruitment, retention and the support of new doctors

Brenda Leese, Jacky Williams, Roland Petchey, Bonnie Sibbald and Toby Gosden

This chapter describes the origins and early experiences of Personal Medical Services with particular respect to salaried general practitioners and the impact on GP recruitment.

The policy background

During the 1990s, primary care has undergone a series of organisational changes, including the introduction of GP fundholding[1] and its extension to total purchasing,[2] multifunds, commissioning groups,[3] Personal Medical Services (PMS),[4] and primary care groups (PCGs)[5] and trusts (PCTs). Since the start of the NHS in 1948, GPs have been independent contractors, undertaking to provide general medical services (GMS) for the patients on their list as part of their contract with the NHS. This national contract was extensively reformed in 1990 to introduce greater accountability of GPs. Remuneration for GPs has four elements – capitation, allowances, target payments and fee for service – set out in the Red Book[6] and renegotiated annually.

PMS pilots arose out of the 1997 NHS (Primary Care) Act[7,8] which concluded that the national GP contract was not sufficiently sensitive to address health inequalities and had insufficient flexibility to provide the necessary employment opportunities for GPs, particularly in deprived areas.[9] The Act coincided with an incoming Labour government which was opposed to the existing competitive internal market and wished to promote a collaborative system of primary care provision. Consequently, PCGs – groups of practices working together – were introduced in a White Paper[10] in order to promote inclusivity. Although PMS had been introduced by a Conservative government, it was retained by the incoming Labour government, alongside the introduction of PCGs, because it fitted well with the desire to address health inequalities.

PMS would be one way of allowing GPs to do what they like best – practising medicine – by removing much of the burden of administration and encouraging improved recruitment and retention in deprived areas. Under PMS, GP practices, NHS trusts and NHS employees can contract to provide services tailored to serve local needs. This type of PMS contract is undertaken between the pilot and the health authority and sets out the pilot's strategy and objectives. GPs in the pilots provide personal medical services to patients on the pilot list. Where PMS pilots provide opportunities for the employment of salaried GPs, a specific job contract has also to be negotiated between the salaried GP and the employer, setting out the detailed requirements of the post.

What is PMS?

The pilots provide Personal Medical Services (PMS) and are so designated to indicate that services are provided under the NHS (Primary Care) Act, outside the 1990 national contract. PMS pilots must provide all the services usually supplied under GMS by independent contractor GPs. Some pilots, designated PMS+ (comprising 38% of first wave pilots), may offer a wider range of services, including community or secondary care services, in combination with GMS, under a single contract with the health authority.

PMS was first introduced in 1998 with some 87 pilots being set up.[4] This was followed by a second wave of 203 pilots in 1999, and a third wave[11] of more than 1000 pilots in 2001. Third wave pilots have to comply with a new contractual framework specifying in some detail basic service provision.[12] Furthermore, successful PMS pilots are to become a permanent feature from 2002.[13]

The government's aims and objectives of the PMS scheme are set out in Box 10.1.[4] The majority of the initial 87 first wave pilots, most of which went live in April 1998, consisted of single practices.[9] Other options were, however, taken up, including multi-practice pilots and peripatetic GP services supporting a number of local GMS practices. Interest in PMS has increased with subsequent waves. PMS pilots offer GPs the opportunity to be employed on a salaried basis and this option was taken up in 54% of the first wave pilots. A number of potential benefits of PMS have been identified by the Department of Health[11] and are shown in an abbreviated format in Box 10.2. The salaried option for GPs is likely to contribute most to making improvements for professionals and in promoting recruitment and retention of GPs in areas where this is a problem.

Box 10.1 Aims and objectives of PMS

Aim
- To use the new flexibilities to secure improved health outcomes.

Objectives
- To promote high quality services across the country.
- To provide opportunities and incentives for primary care profes-sionals to use their skills to the full.
- To provide more flexible employment opportunities in primary care.

Box 10.2 Potential benefits of PMS

1 *Improving services for patients*
Improving the quality, range and accessibility of services through:
- developing services to meet identified needs
- tackling unmet need by providing: disease-based services, depriva-tion-based services, client-based services
- new models to provide appropriate and necessary care
- improving the quality and access of treatment
- reducing variations in the quality of services
- providing more responsive services.

2 *Making improvements for professionals*
Improving the recruitment, retention, skills, development and flexibility of professionals through:
- providing opportunities for greater co-operation
- offering ways to improve the interface with secondary care
- enhancing teamworking
- extending opportunities for provision of improved services by role enhancement
- offering greater opportunities for more flexible working.

---

3 Making improvements for the NHS in general
Improving the NHS as a whole through:
- pursuit of equity in allocation of and access to resources
- provision of value for money in improved quality of care
- creation of flexible arrangements to improve recruitment and retention
- improving co-operation in planning local services
- helping PCGs to play a full role in health improvement.

GP recruitment and retention

Set against this background of organisational change and the introduction of PMS pilots are the ongoing problems associated with GP recruitment and retention.[14] Although the numbers of GPs entering and leaving the workforce in the 1990s have largely balanced each other,[15] the perception amongst GP leaders is that there is a crisis situation.[16] Workforce problems have generally been confined to some deprived parts of (usually) urban areas, which have traditionally been unable to attract and/or retain sufficient GPs. The reasons why these problems are now seen as acute is that, firstly, early retirement is an increasing trend amongst GPs. Secondly, the cohort of Asian doctors who entered the primary care workforce in the 1960s and 1970s is nearing retirement age and cannot be replaced from the same source, owing to changes in immigration laws.[16] Thirdly, medicine is becoming a female-dominated profession, with over 50% of the medical school intake being women, many of whom are likely to favour part-time working at some point in their careers. Furthermore, hospital medicine is seen as a more popular career choice than general practice for young medical graduates, so exacerbating the problem.

Many established GPs are also unhappy about the extent of the changes that have taken place in general practice since 1990 – increased bureaucracy, increased workload, lack of flexibility, increased patient expectations and poor remuneration.[17] General practice is, therefore, experiencing increasing recruitment and retention problems at both ends of the age spectrum. Table 10.1 sets out the ways in which doctors enter and leave general practice. Inflows depend on doctors trained in UK medical schools choosing general practice, and doctors being recruited from overseas. Outflows, other than retirement at the usual age, include early retirement, which is increasingly the choice of GPs, and other exits of a temporary or permanent nature.[16]

Table 10.1 Inflows and outflows from general practice

Inflows
• Output from UK medical schools.
• European Union doctors vocationally trained in the UK.
• Migration from elsewhere overseas.

Outflows
• Retirement and early retirement.
• Emigration of UK-trained GPs.
• Re-migration of EU and other overseas-trained doctors.
• Temporary exits from the GP workforce.
• Exits from medicine altogether.

Problems associated with a shortage of GPs can be partly alleviated by skill mix changes within practices, allowing other staff (especially nurses) to undertake enhanced roles.[18] Such changes have been taking place gradually over a number of years but are confounded by a reluctance amongst some GPs to 'let go' and by a shortage of nursing professionals.

Various ways of improving the acceptability of general practice have been introduced, with variable levels of success. Some of those incorporating salaried GPs include Career Start in County Durham,[19] 'Parachuting GPs' in Liverpool[20] and the London Implementation Zone Educational Incentives Scheme (LIZEI) in London.[21] These were all local schemes. PMS is a major *national* scheme set up to improve inequalities in GP provision.

The national evaluation and salaried GPs

In 1998 the Department of Health commissioned a three-year study of salaried GPs in the first wave PMS pilots. The study expected to report in late 2001, but some interim findings are discussed here. Provision of a high quality service, accessible to all, requires a committed workforce in sufficient numbers relevant to local needs. The majority of the first wave pilots were located in deprived areas of major conurbations in line with their requirement to improve the quality of primary care and improve access.[22] These are exactly the types of areas experiencing the most acute GP recruitment and retention problems.

Important questions that might be asked are why would GPs want to become salaried and why would PMS pilots want to employ salaried GPs? Some of the answers to these questions are set out in Boxes 10.3 and 10.4.

In PMS pilots, GPs can negotiate their salaried contracts with their employers and may opt to reduce their administrative commitment. Furthermore, PMS salaried contracts may allow GPs greater flexibility in negotiating the number of hours they are expected to work, so tackling another issue of major concern to GPs – high workload. High workload is a particular problem for GPs in deprived areas, many of whom have high lists and little in the way of team support. PMS provides the opportunity for such GPs and/or practices to take on a salaried doctor in response to such problems.

For young doctors, not having to commit themselves to a practice by 'buying in' at an early stage in their careers can be a positive incentive whilst giving them time to 'find their feet', as can the fact that there is no long-term commitment involved. In this way, PMS salaried contracts can contribute to the support of young doctors.

Box 10.3 Why would GPs want to be salaried?

- More flexible working hours.
- Freedom from administration.
- Increased remuneration.
- No 'buying in' to premises requirement.
- Pay stability.
- No long-term commitment.
- Additional benefits, e.g. vehicle mileage.
- Focus on specific aspects of general practice.
- Improved educational opportunities and professional development.
- Escape from partnership problems.
- A gentle introduction for new GPs.

The primary reason why practices might want to take on a salaried GP must be to improve recruitment and retention. There are a number of ways by which this might be achieved. One way is for individual practices, as part of their PMS contract, to directly employ one or more salaried GPs. Another way is for GPs to be employed by community trusts to work across a number of practices in a locality, or to be employed directly by a number of practices which have grouped together as a pilot. Another reason for appointing a salaried GP could be to target specific areas of service provision that are a cause for concern, perhaps because the workforce is insufficient to cope, or to improve services to specific under-privileged groups such as travellers, refugees, rough sleepers and drug users, all of whom are traditionally hard to reach. Finally, salaried GPs could be appointed to ease the pressure on practices with high lists, and/or those serving an area with a particularly high level of need (Box 10.4).

Box 10.4 Why would practices want salaried GPs?

- To improve recruitment and retention.
- To enhance the quality of service provision in under-served areas by targeting specific activities or patient groups.
- To provide additional staff to practices under pressure, e.g. with high lists.

Table 10.2 sets out the different ways in which GPs can be salaried as part of a PMS pilot.[9] Practices might decide to use PMS to recruit an additional GP on a salaried basis rather than as an independent contractor under GMS, especially where recruitment has been particularly difficult. In some cases existing independent contractors have opted to become salaried as their practice has joined the scheme. Reasons why GPs might choose this option include working in a practice experiencing negative equity or which is in a state of collapse, with difficulties finding locums or staff employment problems. Becoming salaried immediately shifts these problems to the employer. Thirdly, PMS might be used to expand the existing level of GP provision, perhaps to focus on specific issues of concern to the pilot.

Table 10.2 PMS salaried GP schemes

Type 1	Salaried GPs recruited to fill practice vacancies.
Type 2	Change in employment status of existing GPs from independent contractor status to salaried GP.
Type 3	Supernumerary GPs employed to expand the general level of GMS service provision, and/or address specific deficits in given areas of service provision.

PMS is not, however, the complete answer to the disincentives for GP work in deprived areas, since some factors are not affected by the salaried option. GPs will still have to work with needy and possibly demanding patients and their practices are likely to be located in areas with poor amenities, which may cause difficulties for their own families. The salaried option does, however, offer the means to 'escape', not so easily available to those independent contractors who have contributed financially to their practice premises.

Has PMS fulfilled its potential?

The national evaluation of the first wave PMS pilot study looking at the impact of the salaried GP option has sought to identify the successes and failures of the scheme as well as its costs. Some of the early findings are set out here.

Analysis of first wave contracts[22,23] held by salaried GPs showed that 48% of employers were trusts and 28% GP practices. In 24% of cases, contracts had not been drawn up when the analysis was undertaken. Employment benefits offered by salaried contracts were generally good. For example, the employer was likely to deal with vehicle mileage costs and out-of-hours cover, and also offered maternity and paid sick leave as well as contributions to the NHS pension scheme. Annual leave specified was generous, ranging from 25 to 41 days. Furthermore, leave for training, education and personal development featured in 65% of contracts. There was, however, little in the contracts concerning performance management. Administrative demands on the post holder were low.

The mean salary offered under PMS was £43 674, compared with an intended average net remuneration (IANR) for independent contractor GPs of £52 600 for 1999. There were, however, wide variations with some (unspecified) salaries being based on trust consultant scales. Lower pay should be offset against increased employment benefits and, in some cases, reduced workload and management responsibilities. Pay is also stable and does not fluctuate in response to practice profits, which may prove attractive to, for example, young GPs starting out in practice. Matching individual requirements to practices is a key factor. The level of salary and associated benefits are, however, key factors for GPs in areas where there are recruitment and retention problems.

Recruitment in PMS pilots has been a modest success, but the situation may well improve as PMS becomes more mainstream and accepted. It is still early days. The quantity and quality of applicants to salaried posts was investigated. It was found that there were an average of 2.8 applicants per post (range 1–16) and a mean of 2.0 interviews per post (range 0–5). These figures compare with a mean of 5.9 applications for urban deprived areas generally, and 8.5 for all areas combined.[24] Applications per post were higher in London than elsewhere, perhaps because GPs there were used to the concept of salaried initiatives. However, despite the small number of applicants, 85% of pilots were satisfied with the quality of their recruits, many of whom were already known to the pilot. This could be a factor in the finding that the median time to recruitment was just six weeks and that 95% of the 63 posts were filled. National data indicate that 63% of vacancies were filled in three months or less and 89% in six months or less.[22] Only 15% of recruits to PMS pilots were former independent contractor GPs. The majority had moved from GP registrar or locum positions.[23]

Contrary to expectations, 66% of the applicants for salaried posts were male, with a median age of 38 years. Male applicants were older than female (43 as compared to 34 years). It is thought likely that female applicants may increase in number in future years as PMS becomes more established and the entrepreneurial males who relish a challenge have moved on.

Job satisfaction is an important factor in determining whether workers stay in post or move on. This has been tested by comparing the job satisfaction and stress of PMS salaried and independent contractor GPs. It was found that salaried GPs were equally as satisfied overall with their job when compared with independent contractor GPs, and they were more satisfied with their remuneration, working hours and the satisfaction they gained from their work. Insufficient practice resources and their working environment and surgery set up were sources of stress for salaried GPs. Salaried GPs experienced less stress compared with independent contractor GPs in a number of factors, such as being on call, worrying about their finances and long working hours. After adjusting the results for possible confounding factors, salaried GPs were more satisfied overall than independent contractors. These findings suggest that salaried contracts offer the potential to improve job satisfaction. However, lack of attention to the concerns noted above will certainly lead to problems with GP retention.

Future developments

What is likely to be a major issue is whether the salaried option eventually becomes the norm for GPs.[13] This topic has already been the subject of much debate amongst senior GPs and their representatives. There is evidence that the initial opposition to PMS and salaried GPs is waning[22] but it is unlikely to disappear until a critical mass has been achieved. Much will, of course, depend on the salary level ultimately seen as realistic (to GP eyes). It is early days yet to decide whether or not PMS has been successful in alleviating GP recruitment and retention problems or in supporting young doctors. It is, however, clear that there are groups of GPs for whom a salary is a tempting option.

There are a number of key questions still to be answered. For example, it is not yet clear whether PMS is draining supplies of GPs who might otherwise have taken up independent contractor posts. Furthermore, if PMS GPs negotiate fewer working hours, it is questionable whether the pool of GPs and the available funding will be sufficient to sustain these developments. It is, therefore, not possible to say with any certainty whether PMS represents value for money. It would be brave of us to predict with any certainty at this stage that a salaried service for GPs is the best way forward, although government policy is encouraging progression in this direction.

Conclusions

The PMS experiment is continuing and it is as yet too early to predict its eventual outcome although it has the potential to influence the recruitment and retention of GPs in under-served areas. It is seen as providing a model for the development of PCG/Ts in some areas. Its eventual success or failure may well depend on PCG/Ts taking PMS on board and on it becoming more widely accepted and understood.[25]

Summary

- Personal Medical Services (PMS) is a national scheme that enables, among other things, the creation of salaried GP posts.
- Early experience shows extensive uptake of PMS schemes and widespread development of salaried posts.
- Recruitment to the posts has been successful.
- It is too early to predict the eventual outcome, but PMS does appear to have the potential to improve recruitment (and retention) of general practitioners.

References

1   Audit Commission (1996) *Briefing on GP Fundholding.* London, HMSO.
2   Mays N, Goodwin N, Malbon G, Leese B, Mahon A and Wyke S (1998) *What are the Achievements of Total Purchasing Pilot Projects in the First Year and How Can They be Explained?* London, King's Fund.
3   Regan EL, Smith JA and Shapiro JA (1999) *First Off the Starting Block: lessons from GP commissioning pilots for PCGs.* Health Services Management Centre, University of Birmingham, Birmingham.
4   NHS Executive (1997) *Personal Medical Services Pilots under the NHS (Primary Care) Act 1997. A comprehensive guide.* HMSO, London.
5   Wilkin D, Gillam S and Leese B (1999) *The National Tracker Survey of Primary Care Groups and Trusts. Progress and challenges 1999/2000.* National Primary Care research and Development Centre, University of Manchester, Manchester.

6   GPC (2000) *Statement of Fees and Allowances Payable to General Medical Practitioners in England and Wales*. General Practices Committee, London.

7   Department of Health (1997) *The NHS (Primary Care) Act 1997*. The Stationery Office, London.

8   Department of Health (1996) *Choice and Opportunity*. Cm 3390. The Stationery Office, London.

9   Leese B, Gosden T, Riley A, Allen L and Campbell S on behalf of the PMS National Evaluation Team (1999) *Setting Out. Piloting innovations in primary care*. National Primary Care Research and Development Centre, University of Manchester, Manchester.

10   Department of Health (1997) *The New NHS: modern, dependable*. Cm 3807. The Stationery Office, London.

11   NHS Executive (2000) *Personal Medical Services Pilots under the NHS (Primary Care) Act 1997. A comprehensive guide* (3e). The Stationery Office, London.

12   NHS Executive (2000) *A Contractual Framework for Personal Medical Services – Third Wave Pilots*. NHSE, London.

13   Department of Health (2000) *The NHS Plan*. Cm 4818-1. The Stationery Office, London, p. 76.

14   Leese B and Young R (1999) *Disappearing GPs. Debates in Primary Care 3*. National Primary Care Research and Development Centre, University of Manchester, Manchester.

15   Sibbald B, Young R and Leese B (2000) *GP Recruitment and Retention 2. Improving GP recruitment and retention. Executive Summary 19*. National Primary Care Research and Development Centre, University of Manchester, Manchester.

16   Young R and Leese B (1999) Recruitment and retention of general practitioners in the UK: what are the problems and solutions? *British Journal of General Practice*. **49**: 829–33.

17   Sibbald B, Leese B and Young R (2000) *GP Recruitment and Retention 1. Why do GP principals leave practice? Executive Summary 18*. National Primary Care Research and Development Centre, University of Manchester, Manchester.

18   Salvage J and Smith R (2000) Doctors and nurses: doing it differently. *BMJ*. **320**: 1019–20.

19   Harrison J and Redpath L (1998) Career Start in County Durham. In: J Harrison and T van Zwanenberg (eds) *GP Tomorrow*. Radcliffe Medical Press, Oxford.

20   Woodward R, Shridhar S, Dowrick C and May C (1998) Parachuting GPs in the North West. In: J Harrison and T van Zwanenberg (eds) *GP Tomorrow*. Radcliffe Medical Press, Oxford.

21   Freeman G, Fuller J, Hilton S and Smith F (1998) Academic training in London. In: J Harrison and T van Zwanenberg (eds) *GP Tomorrow*. Radcliffe Medical Press, Oxford.

22   The PMS National Evaluation Team (2000) *National Evaluation of the First Wave NHS Personal Medical Services Pilots. Integrated interim report from four research projects*. National Primary Care Research and Development Centre, University of Manchester, Manchester.

23 Williams J, Petchey R, Gosden T, Leese B and Sibbald B (2001) A profile of PMS salaried GP contracts and their impact on recruitment. *Family Practice.* **18**: 283–7.

24 Department of Health (2000) *General Practitioner Recruitment, Retention and Vacancy Survey 2000 for England and Wales.* The Stationery Office, London.

25 General Practitioners' Committee (2000) *An Introduction to Personal Medical Services.* GPC, London.

CHAPTER 11

Helping GPs reflect in mid-career

Virginia Morley

This chapter illustrates a variety of initiatives responding to the needs of pressurised GPs in mid-career. Younger GPs were involved in providing practical support to practices and working in the academic department.

Introduction

The realisation that doctors experience stress at work is not new.[1,2] Such work-related stress for GPs is clearly multidimensional in origin, arising as it does from a number of sources and impinging on the individual doctor in different ways.[3] Indeed, there would seem to be links between an individual's approach to self-criticism which is a strong predictor of stress and work stressors, such as tiredness.[4]

The main source of stress for GPs is workload, especially the effect on personal life. Other sources of stress are organisational change, poor management and insufficient resources to do the job, dealing with patients' suffering, mistakes, complaints and litigation.[5]

Hannay[6] reported a significant increase in general medical services workload following the introduction of the GP contract in 1990, mainly due to more people being seen in clinics with no change in the time spent per patient. Government-initiated changes, such as fundholding, produced competition between practices. In many places these changes did not engender the wished-for closer working between consultants and their GP colleagues. The resulting lack of confidence about what the next change would be, how it might affect them and their position within the NHS also left many GPs confused and uncertain. It can also be argued that since 1990 the climate of continued change directed by successive governments has produced additional pressure for all those working in the NHS.

These changes were also taking place at a time when social service budgets were being cut, thereby reducing support systems for vulnerable and sick people. Many such people found the door to general practice and primary care one of the few left open to them.

When the internal market was abolished under changes initiated by the incoming Labour government in 1997, some anticipated that a calmer time may lie ahead. What emerged following the 1997 White Paper *The New NHS*,[7] was quite different. This was succeeded by a revolution in approach within the NHS to quality and accountability and was fuelled by highly publicised NHS 'crises'. For some, the NHS Plan 2000 has been seen as offering further stress for professionals leading the BMA to canvass doctors about potential mass resignation.

The combination of perceived low morale in GPs and expressed concerns about an ever-increasing and complex workload for existing GP principals in the Lambeth, Southwark and Lewisham area of South London led to the idea of developing a Mid-Career Break Scheme (MCBS).

The Mid-Career Break Scheme

The Mid Career Break Scheme (MCBS) 1996-1999 gave GP principals aged 37–55:

- the opportunity to take part in a number of specifically designed education and learning opportunities
- the chance to continue their professional development
- a place to refresh and maintain their interest and enthusiasm for general practice and primary care in South London.

This was achieved by:

- initial focus groups – offering GPs an opportunity to take part in the design and structure of the MCBS
- a series of mid-career review seminars – offering GPs career review opportunities to allow them time to reflect on their careers and plan for the future both individually and in a peer group
- 'Take a Break' – a one-day-a-week programme combining an 'action learning set' with time to develop a project for six months; organised GP assistant/research associate cover was provided for GPs taking time out

- 'Time for a Change' – a two-and-a-half-day-a-week programme combining an 'action learning set' with a more substantial period of time to develop a project; organised GP assistant/research associate cover was also provided to the practice where the GP took time out.

At the outset, the scheme was committed to taking GPs who reflected the broad range of practitioners working locally. The focus was therefore not on those who were already part of the so-called 'innovator' group – what has been described as the 'leading edge'. Nor did we wish to take GPs who would be unable to cope with the group interventions proposed or for whom the project would be inappropriate. Our interest was primarily in GPs between the two extremes of performance and during the middle years of their careers.

Focus groups

In Spring 1996, groups of GPs were invited to take part in three focus groups to consider how the development of the MCBS could best meet their needs. GPs were randomly selected from the health authority list, to include a range of men and women from different parts of the area, large and small practices and different ethnic backgrounds.

While they were very interested in developing new skills, there was considerable enthusiasm for taking time out of the practice to reflect on their current work, especially since workload seemed to be a problem. This time for reflection would allow the opportunity to 'think about the next ten years' and to 'get off the treadmill' (Box 11.1). It was seen as an opportunity to energise and refresh their sense of what general practice was about and to put their career into perspective.

Box 11.1 Perceived benefits for GPs in taking part in mid-career breaks

- Using computers more effectively.
- Developing management capabilities.
- Reviewing clinical knowledge.
- Learning minor surgical techniques such as injecting joints.
- Understanding complementary medicine.
- Pursuing managerial issues such as commissioning.

It was hoped that the MCBS would be an opportunity for personal and professional development. Creating a self-directed learning programme within the structure of a peer group setting looked attractive. Meeting local colleagues would provide the opportunity for peer support within a group, thereby reducing isolation; different practices would be represented, so that a network of mutual interest could be built up over time; and they would learn from each other.

In order to feel able to take part in the scheme, the GPs in mid-career had a number of requirements. From their point of view, the scheme needed to:

- provide high quality, consistent clinical cover
- be tailored to meet the needs of the individual, who would then be motivated to make best use of the time
- be of visible gain, not only to the existing GP partner taking the time out, but also to the practice and patients
- be considered a 'long-term' development, offering all GPs locally an opportunity to take part
- offer something 'different' which would provide a new sense of satisfaction – something separate from their day-to-day work.

GPs were asked to consider what would be difficult about taking part in a career break. There were fears and anxieties about leaving behind a job of work that still needed to be done, combined with uncertainties about what the career break might hold in store and how this might affect them.

There were worries about being seen to place a further burden on the partners left behind; dealing with the envy of partners; and partnerships described as 'going into freeze until I get back'.

Other issues raised included making the decision to do it: 'What would I have to give up to do it?'; 'My own development has taken low priority'; 'Making the choice to do it.' There were concerns about fitting it all in: 'Guilt about being a working mother, about general practice, about families.' There were also fears about what would happen to them during their time out: 'It might plant seeds of dissatisfaction'; 'Getting started is easy, finishing may be more difficult.'

Mid-career review seminars

Throughout the life of the MCBS the scheme ran two-day residential events. These were intended as taster events for the larger programmes as well as events in their own right. Following on from these a number of GPs also took up other educational opportunities available through the London Initiative Zone Educational Incentives (LIZ EI) funding outside of the MCBS.

During the seminars the GPs expressed concerns about:

- perceived changes in the core value system associated with general practice

- difficulties in relationships with the health authority
- the changing nature of the doctor–patient relationship, in particular with respect to complaints
- limited support networks.

Many of these themes also emerged in action learning sets in 'Take a Break' and 'Time for a Change'. GPs also commented that the seminars were most useful in providing a forum in which particular personal problems were identified and explored, leading hopefully to resolution:

> An opportunity to look at real conflicts, issues and problems of myself, others and the practice.

> Looking at the future – helped to identify personal priorities.

> Hearing others' experience stimulated lots of new ideas and ways of implementing them.

> Small groups very supportive in validating and encouraging ideas.

> Looking at areas of support.

> Possibilities of reducing stress in the practice and reassessing what positive action could be taken.

'Take a Break'

This programme ran four times between October 1996 and March 1999. The programme was oversubscribed and, in total, 31 GPs took part.

Table 11.1 GPs taking part in MCBS, Oct 1996–April 1999

Programme	Total no. applicants	Total no. particip- ants	Male	Female	Age range	Average age	Single- handed	Group practice
Take a Break 1 Oct 96–Apr 97	10	8	4	4	37–56	45	3	5
Take a Break 2 May 97–Oct 97	30	7	3	4	39–53	44	1	6
Take a Break 3 Nov 97–Apr 98	15	8	5	3	37–54	44	1	7
Take a Break 98* Oct 98–Apr 99	11	8	4	4	37–54	45	1	7
	66	31	16	15			6	25

* NB: Programme started after end of LIZ EI in October 1998.

The programme included:

- one day a week of protected time out over six months
- a two-day residential programme at the beginning
- an 'action learning set' of peers as a core component to encourage GPs to learn new approaches to problem solving in relation to their work setting
- a supervised project of their choice.

> A typical action learning set is a small learning group which meets periodically over a drawn-out period of time, allowing space for action between meetings. At meetings each person in turn is offered space and time to consider what they might do next in the light of their experiences since the set last met.[8]

The action learning set model of group work was chosen to fit with GPs' expressed needs, offering an approach which linked work experiences and problem solving.

Each of the action learning sets contained a mix of male and female GPs aged 37–55 from practices of different sizes across South London. Access to the programme was through written application and interview. The problems addressed were clinical, organisational, professional and personal. Practical and emotional support was provided. The issues of stress and increasing workload arose repeatedly. A common understanding of these issues and how they affect individual GPs was shared. The perceived overload in service commitment and what this means to the practice and at what cost at a personal level was also a frequent topic of discussion.

Other topics discussed related to practice work, particularly relationships with partners, challenges in communication, and management and staffing issues.

At a personal level, GPs spent time reviewing support mechanisms for staying in practice and exploring ways of maintaining the 'space' released through the 'Take a Break' programme.

'Time for a Change'

This substantial intervention allowed an individual GP to take time out of practice for two and a half days a week and provided three days of GP assistant/research associate cover in the practice. The first group of four participants ran from April to October 1997, with a second group of five GPs starting in November 1997 and running to May 1998.

Table 11.2 GPs taking part in MCBS, May 1997–April 1998

Programme	Total no. applicants	Total no. participants	Male	Female	Age range	Average age	Single-handed	Group practice
Time for a Change 1 May 97–Oct 97	11	4	3	1	38–51	41	1	3
Time for a Change 2 Nov 97–Apr 98	8	5	3	2	40–50	43	0	5
	19	9	6	3			1	8

Access to the programme was by application and interview. In contrast to the 'Take a Break' programme, applicants had to demonstrate a significant understanding of how they would plan to undertake their project. The programme was similar in design to 'Take a Break' in that it involved a weekly action learning set and provided project supervision and support. Wherever possible, applicants were sought who reflected the variety of local practices.

Supervision in the initial phases of the project helped to clarify objectives, give realistic boundaries and develop project management skills. Help was provided in carrying out literature searches and in methodology.

The action learning sets reserved some of their time for individual problem solving, as well as allowing space for review and topic presentation.

Overall, they explored the kind of practitioners they hoped to become, their underlying ideals, and the realities and disappointments of general practice as they experienced it. While some groups ended with the programme, others continued to meet on an ongoing basis with an external facilitator, funded by the GPs and in their own time.

Under supervision, participants have undertaken a wide range of different and contrasting projects including those listed in Box 11.2.

Box 11.2 Projects undertaken by participants on the Mid-Career Break Scheme

- Developing personal assertiveness.
- Locality commissioning and fundholding.
- Assessing and modifying a tool to make GPs' databases compatible.
- Survey of local pharmacists.
- Making improvements to the mental health of deprived populations.
- Length of time taken to receive emergency treatment.
- Developing working relationships with local hospital-based geriatricians.

- Developing facilitation skills.
- Practice management issues and change.
- Leadership principles applied to a GP practice.
- Sports medicine course.
- Needs assessment process to target resources more effectively.
- Developing IT skills.
- Study for MRCGP.
- Using IT to aid the thinking process in the consultation.
- Updating in clinical issues.
- Researching the history of penicillin.
- Developing skills to give parents better advice.
- Support for GPs who are improving their premises.
- Enhancing the skills of practice nurses and their use of time.
- Improving an understanding of locality commissioning and its implications for general practice.
- Occupational health.
- Dermatology.
- Acupuncture.
- Handling emotion in consultation (a GP's perspective).
- Interpersonal dynamics of groups.
- Developing a new partnership.

The funding for the MCBS ended in Spring 1999 with little in prospect to continue the programmes we had started. Our main focus therefore, shifted towards the six primary care groups (PCGs) locally supporting the continuation of the now well-established GP assistant/research associate scheme which had been part of the essential underpinning of the MCBS. This new scheme supported time out for GPs taking up their new roles on PCG boards and for placing GP assistants/research associates in practices where there was a known difficulty, e.g. death of a partner, recent partnership split, premises difficulties. A requirement for all established GPs receiving GP assistant time was to take part in an action learning set, which met monthly over the nine months.

This scheme was evaluated during 1999–2000 and five key findings emerged: enthusiastic support for the continuation of the scheme; GPAs' personal and professional development (new knowledge/eye openers/ managing multiple roles/feeling vulnerable/time constraints/empowering processes); challenges for managing the scheme; need for greater co-operation and collaborative working; recognition of the scheme within a career pathway for general practice.[9]

GP assistants/research associates

GPs locally continue to emphasise the need for high quality doctor cover to be organised and available if they are to take part in any scheme like the MCBS. GP assistants/research associates have been recruited now since 1996, working up to seven clinical sessions in one or more practices to provide this. Their remaining sessions have been spent in the academic department of general practice and primary care undertaking teaching, research and development. Offering a flexible working and supported environment to the individuals taking up these posts has clearly been important in attracting high quality young practitioners to the scheme.

The 21 GP assistants/research associates who took up these posts varied in age from 30 to 43 and had worked in general practice for less than five years.

Mentoring and project supervision from the academic department supported their development, encouraging them to work in areas where the department already had recognised strengths. GP assistant/research associates have worked in a specific area within the department, reflecting the wide range of individual interests, including those listed in Table 11.3.

All GP assistants/research associates developed new skills, enhancing the work of the department, whether it be in supervised research or teaching

Table 11.3 The GP assistant/research associates working on the MCBS Oct 96–April 99 projects

- Access to out-of-hours healthcare services
- Asthma research
- Chronic illness: heart failure
- Community Trust undergraduate education project
- Computer assisted learning
- Computer assisted learning in medical ethics
- Continuing care in general practice
- Developing and research into consulting patterns
- Developing and research into field of social exclusion and inequality
- Developing writing skills (ethics)
- Development of joint disease register for patients with mental health illness
- Emergency medical care, immediate access research and development/out-of-hours
- Identifying a database of websites relevant to healthcare professionals and community staff
- Immediate access research and development/out-of-hours
- Management in general practice
- Multiprofessional audit research
- Planning for long-term community study
- Postgraduate education
- Undergraduate teaching, chronic illness

and development. It could be argued that this group of GP assistants/ research associates represents a way forward for expanding the range of opportunities available for academic training in general practice and primary care. The scheme has now developed as a separate stream of activity and, in 1999–2001, there were 17 GP assistants/research associates working in the department. This work is being further strengthened and GP assistants/research associates will be offered the opportunity to undertake an MSc in general practice during their time in the department. An approach to joint recruitment of young GPs locally has also just started with advertising and recruitment for Vocationally Trained Associates (VTAs), GP assistants/research associates and Personal Medical Services (PMS) posts.

At the beginning of their time in post, a weekly peer support group for the GP assistants/research associates was set up. The group was externally facilitated and has varied in size as the programme has expanded.

At the beginning of each group the GP assistants/research associates identify a number of aims for the group which have included the following:

- reflecting on their clinical work and research
- thinking about their futures
- discussing specific clinical issues
- exploring broader issues such as the White Paper on primary care
- discussing the 'nuts and bolts' of the practices in which they worked
- having individual 'slots' to talk about the past week.

General practitioners at mid-career

The work with GPs as professionals at the mid-point of their career has been and is developing. However, a number of themes have emerged which seem core to the successful development of such programmes.

Attracting and enabling GPs to participate

The very idea of a mid-career break was, and continues to be, judging by the adaptation of the scheme beyond 1999, appealing to a number of GPs who feel under considerable pressure and at times consider leaving general practice altogether.

Developing a scheme to refresh and re-energise these practitioners was our task and some of the key elements for this were:

- attracting sufficient interest and confidence from funders, whether health authority, PCG or now primary care trust, to make substantial investment in practitioners and practices where there are and may be ongoing difficulties
- making application to the scheme easy for GPs, who often perceive hurdles such as application and interview daunting
- facilitating an action learning set
- providing the opportunity to develop individual interests
- giving consistent and high quality clinical support to practices to enable GPs to be released
- encouraging and promoting a model of professional and personal development for GPs which they may not be familiar with.

At the outset, some GPs on the programme were concerned about being labelled as those 'who can't cope'. The success of the programme meant this diminished rapidly over time. Equally though GPs can find it hard to ask for help. There are opportunities to intervene before GPs experience burnout, but recognising the need for personal and professional development or knowing what to ask for may not be easy for those most at risk.

Easing communication with GPs has been an important part of the scheme, particularly in explaining the scheme, how it works and its limitations. Even so, communication continues to be a challenge. Dealing with anxious GPs, unused to writing about or clearly stating their needs, presents not insignificant organisational hurdles.

The action learning set approach

At the outset we were clear that important aspects of any career break should be:

- to address work-related problems
- to reduce the reported professional and social isolation experienced by many GPs
- to develop interpersonal networks.

GPs said they wanted to meet colleagues, to share ideas and to discuss different ways of doing things in practice. The action learning sets have clearly been invaluable to many GPs who have seen them as crucial to promoting positive changes in themselves.

Working in partnerships

Feeling 'overloaded with work' and the pressures of caring for patients have been persistent themes of discussion in the action learning sets. This has not lessened over the time we have been working in this area. In many instances, it could be said to have increased as lines of accountability changed, first for GPs from the health authority to PCGs, and now again to PCTs configured with different personnel, boundaries and organisational culture.

Working in partnerships, where patterns of behaviour become fixed and difficult to change, has also been an important issue for discussion. It was revealing to find that many established GPs now see a model of partnership as inappropriate, much as young GPs do, and the rapid rise in the number of PMS practices locally may reflect this. Continuous clinical responsibility, fears of being exploited and commitment to working in one place with perhaps only two or three colleagues over a lifetime no longer seems attractive.

What about those not in mid-career?

The defined age group of 37–55 years is not an unreasonable definition of mid-career. However, should the aim be to support all GPs by stimulating ongoing professional and personal development? Then five-yearly career breaks could be viewed as appropriate for all practitioners, not just for those in mid-career. At the moment the GP assistant/research associate scheme offers young salaried GPs a peer group with a facilitator and this is considered essential.

It is now evident that peer support groups should be available to all GPs should they wish to take part, whether having just entered practice and learning to understand the pressures of clinical care and the dynamics of practice life, or whether a practitioner is later on in her/his career and considering succession planning and retirement.

Taking back control

We are aware of the following individual actions following on from the 'Take a Break' and 'Time for a Change' programmes:

- changing future career plans, including options for part-time working and/or taking on new roles in the workplace

- ensuring continued space in the working week for reflection
- renegotiating partnership arrangements
- continued membership of an action learning set
- planning future education and training, meeting with outside agencies with a view to developing different working patterns
- a number of GPs from these programmes taking up board-level posts in PCGs.

In addition, we have learned how difficult it is for established GPs to change later in their career. Some of the reasons for this may be

- the unrelenting daily pressure of coping with routine work
- professional commitment to patient care
- the limited mechanisms present to support changes
- the relatively isolating structure of general practice
- the extent of family and financial commitments.

Relieving stress

An important part of the mid-career break scheme evaluation was to gather data about different dimensions of the GP participants' life and practice. Questionnaires applied before and after the programme in 1996–7 included the occupational stress indicator, the GP attitude questionnaire, the general wellbeing survey and an inner-city practice questionnaire.

At the start of the 'Take a Break' programme, GPs expressed feelings of stress over:

- participation in decision making
- flexibility (or lack of it) in their working lives
- dealing with change
- implementing policies
- communication
- personal relationships at work.

The range of perceived stress was wide but most was experienced as a result of high workload, rising patient expectations and what were felt to be unreasonable demands from patients. High workload was felt to be due to problems related to unemployment, poverty, mental health and an ageing population.

Analysis of questionnaires suggested that, by the end of the 'Take a Break' programme 1996–7, the perception of general practice as a stressful job, the extent of such stress and ideas about the sources from which stress comes were unchanged.

However, coping skills to reduce potential stress and enhance job satisfaction and physical health had all improved.

Techniques to reduce feelings of stress included:

- using logical thought processes to deal with problems
- using the home environment as a support
- developing interests outside medicine.

Participants reported improved job satisfaction, resulting from decreased feelings of frustration with the policies and characteristics of the organisations in which they worked. There was also increased pleasure in relationships with colleagues and with the atmosphere in the practice.

Comment

The overt politicisation of the NHS and the climate of continuous change mean that stress has now become an almost inevitable component of modern general practice and primary care.

The recent move to Personal Medical Services (PMS) contracts which has been welcomed and taken up in South London has been used positively to enable doctors who do not aspire to traditional models of partnership to work in general practice. This, allied to the introduction of primary care trusts which offers more opportunities for salaried GPs, suggests new models of employment for general practitioners will continue to emerge.

The drive for quality allied to the necessarily bureaucratic requirements of accountability are likely to continue to present GPs with ongoing challenges. To counteract this the belated advent of protected learning time is now becoming accepted at all levels within the NHS. The time for reflection, evaluation and planning which the schemes describe within this chapter could become more widely available.

One barrier for time out for GPs in mid-career may also be the unavailability of prolonged study leave as a right for PMS GPs in contrast with those still employed under GMS contracts. It is to be hoped that PCTs and health authorities have the vision to develop this opportunity.

The projects detailed in this chapter also give support to the principles underlying PMS – that innovation and imagination can be employed successfully to recruit young GPs into primary care. The continuing success of recruitment to assistant programmes as demonstrated recently with attachments to an academic department and the MSc course provide a lead in showing how inner London can continue to recruit high quality young GPs committed to providing a service.

As the new century develops, recruitment schemes for attracting these young GPs and projects which provide for established GPs to reflect and refresh themselves seem likely to be an important aspect of primary care development.

Summary

- GPs in mid-career face many demands.
- A Mid-Career Break Scheme offers a variety of options for professional and personal development.
- Career reflection can lead to planned changes.
- GPs can regain career control with support.
- Skills for coping with stress can be improved.
- High quality, consistent GP cover is essential to implement change and participate in such schemes.
- Peer support is vital.
- Similar interventions to those for GPs at mid-career may be appropriate both earlier and later in GPs' careers.

Acknowledgements

The development of the Mid-Career Break Scheme was based on an idea by Professor Roger Higgs. Its progress into the GP assistant/research associate scheme has depended on the continued support and funding of Lambeth, Southwark and Lewisham Health Authority and the primary care groups locally.

The continuing professional development team involves a range of individuals who contribute both to the dynamic nature of the scheme and to its overall success and evaluation. I should therefore like to thank and acknowledge all the GPs who have taken part, the GP assistants/research associates, Annie Atherton, Christine Bell, Loretta Bellman, Helen Cork, Annette Cox, Tim Dartington, Tony Emerson, Lesley Higgins, Roger Higgs, Roger Jones, Lisl Klein, Priscilla Laurence, Faruk Majid, Monica Martin, Jan McHugh, Fran Ross, Tricia Scott, John Seex, Nicki Speigal, Alison Wertheimer, Patrick White and Paul Woodgate.

References

1   Quill T and Williamson P (1990) Healthy approaches to physician stress. *Archives of Internal Medicine.* **150**: 1857–61.

2   Johnson W (1991) Predisposition to emotional distress and psychiatric illness amongst doctors: the role of unconscious and experiential factors. *British Journal of Medical Psychology.* **64**: 317–29.

3   Firth Cozens J (1998) Individual and organisational predictors of depression in general practitioners. *British Journal of General Practic.* **48**: 1647–51.

4   Firth Cozens J (1997) Predicting stress in general practitioners: 10 year follow up postal survey. *BMJ.* **315**: 34–5; BMA (2000) *Report on Work Related Stress among Senior Doctors.* British Medical Association, London.

6   Hannay D, Usherwood T and Platts M (1992) Workload of general practitioners before and after the new contract. *BMJ.* **304**: 615–18.

7   Department of Health (1997) *The New NHS: modern, dependable.* The Stationery Office, London.

8   Casey D (1996) *Managing Learning in Organisations.* Open University, Buckingham.

9   Bellman L and Morley V (2001) *GPs in Transition – The GP Assistant/Research Associate Scheme.* Bayswater Institute/Guy's, King's and St Thomas' School of Medicine, London.

CHAPTER 12

Rural general practice

Iain Mungall and John Gillies

I have no relish for the country; it is a kind of healthy grave.
Sydney Smith

> This chapter explores issues facing rural GPs and highlights recent initiatives in rural networking and co-operation

Rural practice cannot escape post-modernism. For example, over the past few decades, the population of many rural areas has changed from a local population expressing itself through an indigenous monoculture to an eclectic mix of cultures, as many 'outsiders' are attracted to the pleasures of rural life. In addition, there are major issues to be addressed in recruitment and retention, in adapting training and continuing professional development (CPD) to the extended role of the rural doctor, in organising out-of-hours care that provides a quality service for patients and adequate time off for GPs, in achieving equity of provision for rural populations, in putting rural issues on the research agenda and in using the powerful new tools of information technology to best effect. There are many new developments in all these areas which suggest good cause for optimism about the future.

What is rural practice?

Although few people would have difficulty in recognising a rural area, defining rurality is problematic.[1] Population sparsity and isolation are two major defining components, but firm definitions are elusive and probably only necessary for academic work. There is obviously a continuum of rurality from practice in near suburbia to practice in the remote islands of Orkney, Shetland and the Hebrides.

Rural practices tend to be small and isolated; there is reduced opportunity for division of labour and more clinical skills may be required for trauma, acute medical and obstetric care. Professional isolation is a potential problem both because of the difficulties of meeting with colleagues on a regular basis, and also for continuing professional development.

Health of rural dwellers

In broad terms, rural dwellers are healthier than urban dwellers, with lower mortality rates, though these rates increase in more remote areas. However, some northern rural areas have higher mortality rates than some southern urban areas. Mortality from trauma, especially road and farm accidents, is higher amongst rural residents.

Morbidity rates can be related to distance from care, and some studies show late presentation of disease correlating with remoteness.

Access to care

This is a major issue. Although not all of the contributing factors have yet been well defined, there is good evidence that the distance away from both primary and secondary care affects the uptake of services by patients with consequent effects on health. A recent study[2] suggested that distance from a cancer centre was associated with less chance of diagnosis before death for stomach, breast and colorectal cancers, and poorer survival after diagnosis for lung and prostate cancer.

Many patients with cancer requiring chemotherapy or radiotherapy spend a considerable part of their last months travelling to distant hospitals for treatment.[3] Pilot studies suggest that telemedicine developments have promise in this area.[4] Naturally those without ready access to transport are most disadvantaged, particularly young families, the poor and the elderly. There may also be difficulties for young people who require contraception or information on sexual health in approaching local GPs or nurses.

In the last two years, government has emphasised the importance of access to care, although, to date, this has been largely from an urban perspective, and problems of geographic access have scarcely been addressed: it is left up to individual practices to decide how accessible their services should be. Some rural practices have branch surgeries of varying sophistication, and some practices have higher-than-average visiting rates in an attempt to cope with difficulties in access to care, although this tends to be at some personal cost to the practice. Here a real dilemma is introduced, since it is likely that the standard of care on offer at branch surgeries is not as high as that on offer at the main surgeries, due to difficulties with access to notes and to other members of the practice team. There has been a trend over recent years to close down branch surgeries, but there is little evidence as to whether or not this has affected patients' health.

Community hospitals

In many rural areas, these GP-led units offer acute medical care, day hospital services, rehabilitation, assessment and sometimes obstetric care near to the patient's home. They avoid the difficulties and risks of travelling long distances for patients and relatives, who are often elderly. There are major issues around staffing and payment for GPs providing these services, but they are popular with GPs and patients, and are an under-utilised teaching resource.[5] A recent review offers an optimistic assessment for the future, but current resource constraints threaten the future of many community hospitals.[6]

Maternity care

Home births are dramatically less frequent than a generation ago. However, for isolated communities the opportunity to deliver at home or in a nearby community hospital is much appreciated, and the evidence shows that, when carefully selected, many women can deliver their babies in safety away from a 'high tech' district general hospital. However, at least 5% of women will have unpredicted problems during childbirth, so the professional needs sufficient training and resources to be able to manage the unexpected.[7]

Deprivation

Phillimore and Reading showed that illness was closely related to deprivation, and that matched studies for those similarly deprived showed no difference in health with geographic setting.[8]

Although deprivation tends to be thought of as an urban phenomenon, rural deprivation exists but is more hidden. Classically, the large country mansion houses its workers at the back in tied accommodation of poor quality. Traditional indices of deprivation tend not to identify the small pockets of rural deprivation. For example, ethnic populations and car owner-ship are not valid pointers in most UK rural areas. The Rural Voice Health Group has listed indicators of rural deprivation;[9] and the RCGP Rural Doctors Group is endeavouring to find a measure of this rural deprivation, to help target resources to the appropriate areas. Work undertaken in Northern Ireland by PricewaterhouseCoopers has developed a formula to identify equitable resourcing across differing rural areas, particularly in the field of community nursing.[10]

Rural illness and disease

Some diseases or problems are peculiar to or more prevalent in rural areas. Arthritis of the hip is very common in agricultural workers[11] and suicide rates are higher than average amongst farmers. The culture of farming communities may make it difficult for individuals to seek and receive help during difficult personal or financial circumstances.[12] Many rural GPs will provide a first-contact casualty service and will often deal with most minor trauma. They are also often involved in local BASICS organisations and deal with the major trauma of road traffic and farming accidents.[13] Geography means that in remote areas, they are often at the scene of accidents before ambulance paramedics.

Agricultural workers are at risk of farmer's lung and organic toxic dust. Rural dwellers are at increased risk from zoonoses, e.g. Orf and Lyme disease, because of their contact with animals, either directly or through private water supplies or water-based recreation.[14]

In rural areas, more patients die at home than in urban areas, and geography dictates that more palliative and terminal care is undertaken at home.[15]

Some issues for rural practices

Recruitment

Rural practice has shared in the decline in numbers of GP registrars over the past five years and it is now apparent that there are many vocationally trained GPs who choose not to enter general practice as principals.[16] A recent survey revealed that in Scotland there are a disproportionate number of vacant rural registrar places (20% urban vacancies, compared to 30% rural vacancies).[17] Many more rural registrars were from mainland Europe, and only 20% of all registrars wished to find a principal post immediately on completing training. The main addressable factors deterring registrars from pursuing a career in rural practice were on-call issues, professional isolation and the degree of clinical responsibility for which they felt untrained. The inflexible nature of the GP career structure was a deterrent to many. It is essential that these factors be addressed in future workforce planning if a crisis in GP provision in rural areas, already a reality in many countries, is to be averted. The positive rewards of a career in rural practice also need to be highlighted.[18]

To that end, the recent WONCA policy document *Policy for Training for Rural Practice*[19] suggests a co-ordinated approach to improving recruitment and enhancing rural training. Ideas include measures to increase the numbers of students recruited from rural areas, increasing exposure to rural practice in the undergraduate curriculum, tailored rural vocational training to reflect the increased clinical responsibilities of rural practice, developing academic positions for rural doctors, and measures to improve on call and support the rural doctor's family.

Resourcing

The costs of providing optimum standards of care in different geographical settings have, unbelievably, not been measured; however, it seems likely that these costs are higher in rural areas.

Specific funding for rural general practice comes from:

- rural practice payments, (a capitation-based mileage payment scheme)
- profits from dispensing (not available for all rural practices, and widely seen as under threat)
- for a few practices, the inducement scheme (to provide a guaranteed minimum income for practices with very low populations).

This funding compensates for:

- low practice populations, with few opportunities to expand list sizes
- lack of non-general medical services work
- travelling costs, and sometimes the need for four-wheel-drive transport
- extra costs for communications
- lack of economies of scale
- accident and emergency and Immediate Care Scheme work
- other work undertaken because of the distance from secondary care.

As the work involved, and the associated costs for this, will vary greatly in different rural settings, there is often little correlation between the actual expenditure and the reimbursement. Following a major study of rural practices in the north of England, Rousseau and McColl noted that 'it is unlikely that the amount of indirectly reimbursed expenditure will equate, except by chance, to actual expenditure,' and recommended that the particular problems of GPs in areas remote from secondary care should be given greater recognition.[20]

The RCGP Rural Doctors Group has recommended that adequate reimbursement of the true expenses of rural practices should be separated from the ability to dispense, and a case for doctor dispensing could then be argued on its merits.

Personal Medical Services (PMS)

The development of PMS as an alternative to the historical GMS contract for GPs, may allow local needs to be addressed more sensitively in rural areas; yet it remains unclear to what extent contracts will be centrally determined. Political drivers are moving this agenda forward, with ambitious targets for expansion of PMS over the next few years.

Communication/information technology

Covering a large area means inevitably a considerable length of time is spent travelling, so keeping in touch is a major problem. Increasingly, mobile phones are covering the vast majority of the UK. However, invariably the areas of inadequate coverage are sparsely populated rural areas! Message bleeps and VHF radios frequently have better coverage than mobile telephones; it is likely that satellite telephones will become more widely available and affordable in the near future.

Telemedicine

This has been piloted around the country and has been shown to be useful for linking GPs with consultants, who can, via a remote video consultation, share a clear view of, for example, a skin lesion or an ECG recording, and advise on management of the patient. Prevention of unnecessary patient travelling, improving interprofessional relationships and learning at the same time are potential benefits, but the true costs and benefits are yet to be established. A recent review suggests that there is evidence that health services can be successfully and effectively delivered to isolated communities by telemedicine, but much of it relates to work done outside the UK. This should be taken into account in future strategic health planning for the UK.[21,22]

Out-of-hours provision

The allocation in 1995 of additional funding to develop innovative means of coping with the out-of-hours service has seen enormous changes in the provision of this part of general practice, particularly the rapidly accelerating development of co-operatives. The majority of GPs now provide an out-of-hours service via a co-operative, normally working shifts from a primary care centre. Most doctors have felt enormous improvements in their quality of life as a result of these changes.

It remains to be seen how far co-operatives can spread into remote rural areas. Already they are working successfully in extremely rural parts of the country, e.g. Cornwall, Northumberland, Cumbria, the Scottish Borders and Northern Ireland. However, it seems clear that there must be some limits to this and these as yet have not been defined. Clearly, for example, some remote islands with small populations, e.g. Orkney, Shetland and the Western Isles of Scotland, would have great difficulty working as part of a co-operative because of unacceptable time delays in making visits. A recent Scottish survey[17] suggests that this may be a major issue for recruitment of GPs to very remote rural practices, and if this proves to be the case then special arrangements will need to be made to ensure access to primary healthcare for isolated patients and to safeguard the quality of life of remote doctors.

Co-operatives continue to spread into increasingly rural areas, facilitated by some targeted payments in 1999, although at the time of going to press this appears to have been a one-off payment and there remains a funding problem for provision of out-of-hours services in rural areas.

In October 2000 the Department of Health commissioned an independent review of GP out-of-hours services in England and their report recommended explicit service standards.[23] It seems likely that these will become *de facto* standards throughout the NHS and may well become a useful measure against which resourcing decisions can be made. The report claimed to find no evidence of increased costs of running co-operatives in rural areas, but noted that this may be largely as a result of lack of information and recommended that as soon as possible the appropriate data should be analysed to ensure that resources are targeted appropriately. It seems likely that in the near future the appropriate resourcing will be provided on a regular basis. It is worth reading the report, particularly to see the new quality standards and recommendations.

Co-operatives have only managed to work successfully because of the concomitant shift away from routine out-of-hours visiting and the increasing expectation that, out-of-hours, patients will, when necessary, attend an out-of-hours centre. Many co-operatives have managed to reduce visiting for patients out of hours to approximately 25% of all contacts. Increased attention has been paid to triaging skills, taking a complete history and often offering to see the patient, but not necessarily at his home.

NHS Direct has been operating as pilots within England and is preparing to go nationwide, and in Scotland NHS24 is currently being rolled out. This offers the possibility of government-funded nursing triage, particularly out of hours. It may be of particular significance for rural doctors since, even when they are so remote that they cannot join together in co-operatives, there will at least be the possibility of these patients seeking advice without always having to contact a doctor, and this may reduce the out-of-hours burden. The initial problems with the nurse triage manpower and training will doubtless be resolved.

The Associate Practitioners' Scheme, which began with the 1990 contract, has gone some way to addressing this issue. Recognising the unique problem of single-handed GPs in isolated areas, the scheme enabled a full-time associate to be employed between two single-handed principals.[24] The post is salaried and enables a doctor to experience remote rural practice without making the commitment of becoming a principal. It has been warmly welcomed by principals as a means of resolving their heavy continuous on-call burden, and the difficulty of leaving the practice for education and leave without incurring a financial burden. The scheme has now been extended to allow for part-time and job-sharing posts. However, there are now major difficulties in finding associates in many areas. Negotiations are currently underway to extend this scheme to remote two-person practices. Some GPs continue to express their satisfaction with being on call on a regular basis for a small number of patients, but eventually the market will have to decide whether regular 24-hour commitment is an acceptable part of the work of isolated rural practices.

RARARI

The Remote And Rural Areas Resource Initiative (RARARI) is a new project funded by the NHS in Scotland to develop healthcare services and support for professional staff in remote and rural parts of Scotland, in primary and secondary care. It is led by a director who is a practising rural GP, and aims to develop new clinically appropriate, accessible and sustainable healthcare models in remote and rural areas within available resources where there are shortcomings in service delivery due to difficulties of access by patients.

The aims of RARARI are:

- new models of remote and rural healthcare, such as managed clinical networks and service redesigns
- better knowledge of patient priorities
- better knowledge of care/process outcomes
- a good remote and rural dataset
- remote and rural health as a defined special interest subject
- new models of staff, education and training
- defined core professional skills
- improved professional morale.

The project has new funding and runs for three years from March 2000. It has an informative website (*see* p. 169), and promises to be a model for development of remote and rural healthcare for the rest of UK and Europe.

Rural Fellows

In Scotland, funding from RARARI has facilitated the development of the Rural Fellows scheme, usually taken up for a two-year period after completion of vocational training. The opportunity to be based in a rural practice and to have time for academic study has been much appreciated, and this may be a route to improving recruitment as well as allowing a longer training period for the extended role of the rural general practitioner.

Continuing professional development

Rural GPs have traditionally found great difficulty in obtaining continuing medical education and have, when possible, tended to take an entire week off when they can get a locum, rather than attend the traditional weekly lecture at a postgraduate centre. Exchanging information with colleagues and getting access to medical libraries has been very difficult. However, progress in ICT has made great strides here, particularly since the development of the Internet. There are now discussion groups especially for rural GPs, both within the UK and worldwide. Medical databases worldwide (such as Medline) can be accessed from home or from the practice, and the development of the techniques for evidence-based medicine have made available remote access to high quality literature reviews, such as the Cochrane Library, *Effectiveness Matters* and *Bandolier*, and appraisal journals such as the *ACP Journal Club*.

Access to the Internet has also improved the ability for rural practices to be involved in research with access to statistical tools, and of course the ability to e-mail colleagues and even to have remote conferencing via e-mail as well as by telephone.

This whole spectrum of developments, allowing GPs to access the latest information on any given subject from their practices, has potentially a greatly empowering effect on GPs. There is a pressing need for training in these areas for rural practice teams, but the increasing pace and funding of practice networks and connections to the NHSNet and SHOW (Scottish Health on the Web) has greatly improved this whole area of communication and information. A recent review, however, suggests that there is some way to go towards making these advances accessible to nurses as well as doctors in remote and rural areas.[25]

Some current developments

Recent years have seen medical students undertaking more of their training within general practice, and a significant number are now able to spend a reasonable amount of time working in rural practices.[5] In addition, the past few years have seen the development of many new organisations interested in rural health issues.

RCGP Rural Doctors Group

In 1994 the RCGP formed a rural doctors' group to help recognise, define and address some of the issues of rural practice. The group has commissioned research, organised conferences and helped raise the profile of rural practice. The group produces a regular newsletter, *Country Matters*, which is circulated to all College rural members and other interested parties, and Occasional Paper No. 71, *Rural General Practice in the UK*, has been published.

The aims of the group are:

- to raise the profile of rural practice
- to stimulate research
- to function as a virtual forum.

The group has contributed to all recent RCGP spring conferences. It is developing the concept of a virtual forum for rural doctors, acknowledging that they have special concerns that are not always shared by other doctors within their local faculty area, and recognising the particular problems of communication and sharing concerns with like-minded people. An index of research of relevance particularly to rural practice is being developed, and the group continues to host discussion groups for rural doctors.

The Montgomeryshire Medical Society

In 1979 this society of rural doctors in mid-Wales organised a conference for rural GPs at Gregynog Hall in Powys, and this has since become an established and successful annual conference which has been highly influential in developing links both within the UK and internationally for health professionals interested in rural health issues.

The Institute of Rural Health

This was established in 1997 to address the broadest definition of health in the rural context. It works with individuals and communities, academic bodies and organisations involved in service delivery. It aims to promote health and wellbeing across rural Britain and to ensure that rural communities receive the highest quality healthcare possible.

Its focus is on research, education, conferences, particularly of a multidisciplinary nature, e-health and publications. It hosts an annual conference for rural GPs.

Current initiatives include:

- young persons' health needs
- a project on stress in farming communities
- a series of briefing papers on relevant topics such as zoonoses, farming accidents, etc.
- a Delphi study to help define differences between rural and urban practice.

Institute of Rural Health publications include the following.

Briefing papers

- Dermatology in a rural community.
- Farm accidents in rural areas.

Conference reports

- Youth in rural areas: are we addressing their needs? (1997).
- Tackling rural stress: causes, effects and ways forward (1997).
- Rural health: a matter of equity. Report of the Rural Health Forum Conference (1998).
- Mental health in the countryside (1999).
- Looking forward to rural health: towards sustainable rural health care (1999).

Research reports

- Boulanger S, Deaville J, Randall-Smith J and Wynn-Jones J (1999) *Farm Suicide in Rural Wales: a review of the services in Powys and Ceredigion.* IRH Research Report 3. Institute of Rural Health, Newtown, Powys.
- Boulanger S, Gilman A, Deaville J and Pollock L (1999) *Farmers' Stress Survey – a questionnaire carried out at the Royal Welsh Show into stress factors experienced by farmers.* IRH Research Report 4. Institute of Rural Health, Newtown, Powys.
- Buchan T (2000) *A Cultural and Spatial Analysis of Adolescent Substance Misuse in Rural Wales: lessons from the literature.* IRH Research Report 8. Institute of Rural Health, Newtown, Powys.
- Davies P (2000) *The Causes and Effects of Stress in Farming Communities in East Anglia.* IRH Research Report 7. IRH and The Countryside Agency. Institute of Rural Health, Newtown, Powys.
- Deaville J (1998) *A Study to Obtain a Definition of Rurality and to Investigate the Problems Encountered by Practitioners who Work in Rural Health Settings.* IRH Research Report 1. Institute of Rural Health and School of Nursing and Midwifery, University of Glamorgan.
- Deaville J (1999) *A Report on Preliminary Work into Unrecognised Psychiatric Morbidity in Farmers and Other Occupational Groups.* IRH Research Report 5.
- Wilson L (1998) *A Breath of Fresh Air – a literature review of trends in the epidemiology, treatment and management of childhood asthma.* IRH Research Report 2. Institute of Rural Health, Newtown, Powys.
- Wilson L (1999) *Asthma in Schools – a survey of school teachers' knowledge of, and attitudes to, asthma in children.* IRH Research Report 6. Institute of Rural Health, Newtown, Powys.

The Centre for Health Services Research

This centre at Newcastle University completed important research on rural health issues in 1997, and this included a detailed literature review. Their work has pointed the way towards future research.[20]

The Department of General Practice, Aberdeen University

This has established an interest in rural health issues. Recent research has focused on telemedicine, cancer care in rural areas[2,4] and the use of information technology.

An example of this work is a collaborative project between the department, Grampian University Hospitals Trust and community hospitals in the Grampian region to establish a 'tele' Accident and Emergency service. This was due to be operational in March 2001, and will cover 30 sites over a large rural area of Scotland.

EURIPA

The European Rural and Isolated Practitioners Association was founded in 1997. It aims to help address the health needs of rural communities in Europe and the professional needs of those serving them. Current areas of interest include acting as a voice for rural health issues in Europe, setting up mechanisms for sharing information, skills and knowledge using Internet technology, promoting recruitment and retention of rural health professionals, initiating rural research and setting up links with other professional organisations, e.g. RCGP and WONCA. At the WONCA 2000 conference in Vienna, EURIPA wokshops were held on: emergencies in rural practice; rural health in Eastern Europe; and European rural research. Delegates were present from Wales, Scotland, England, Ireland, Denmark, Finland, Poland, Spain, Portugal, Greece and Eastern Europe. The secretariat is currently based at the Institute for Rural Health in Wales. A moderated newsgroup has been established and a Charter for Rural Practice has also been drafted. More details are available at the IRH website. WONCA (The World Organisation of General Practitioners) held its second international conference on rural practice in Durban, South Africa, in September 1997. It has already published a seminal report on recruitment for rural general practice.[18]

Other resources

The RCGP website began hosting its first discussion group, for rural practice, in 1996.

Rural Healthcare, the first textbook for rural healthcare in the UK, edited by Cox and Mungall, was published by Radcliffe Medical Press in 1998.[26] *The Textbook of Rural Medicine* contains a review of rural medicine in the UK, together with international comparisons.[27]

The Institute of Rural Health at Gregynog in Wales is currently developing a series of modules for health professionals leading to a Diploma in Rural Health Studies. A non-vocational degree course in rural health studies has been running at the University of the Highlands and Islands since 1998, the first such course available in the UK.

Separate development within the NHS

Health is now one of the responsibilities of the regional parliaments and so we are now seeing divergence in developments within the NHS in England, Wales, Scotland and Northern Ireland. It remains to be seen how this will affect rural doctors, although already it is clear that the Scottish Parliament has recognised the particular issues relating to rurality and have allocated significant funding, e.g. into the RARARI initiative. It will be important for UK-wide organisations to monitor developments and try to identify and spread examples of best practice.

Primary care groups and primary care trusts

There remain anxieties that primary care trusts may not pay sufficient heed to the concerns of their minority rural doctors. Although currently contentious, the option to work under Personal Medical Services rather than General Medical Services contracts may allow the flexibility and funding to address the particular needs of rural practices.

The English countryside White Paper

November 2000 saw the publication of the countryside paper for England, *A Fair Deal for Rural England*,[28] outlining the government's thoughts on rural development. This includes a commitment to address issues of transport in remote areas and a commitment to, and funding for, the development of rural health services. However, it is disappointing in its lack of vision for the future of farming in the UK.

Rural health forum

In recent years there has been an annual conference under the auspices of the IRH, the Countryside Agency, Rural Voice and the National Council for Voluntary Agencies which brings together a wide range of interested parties to look at the problems of rural health.

Some useful websites and online groups

- RCGP rural group – www.rcgp.org.uk/special/rural/index.htm
- Institute of Rural Health – www.rural-health.ac.uk
- RARARI – www.rarari.org.uk
- EURIPA mailing list – euripa@onelist.com
- Rural Doctors discussion group – rural.practice@ukpractice.net

Conclusion

Rural practice has long been bedevilled by its isolation and little has been done to define and celebrate its differences, its challenges and its successes. However, the 1990s saw an explosion of interest, research work and literature, which are helping to clarify the issues, and will enable sensible decisions to be made about allocation of resources and efficient and equitable delivery of care right across the country.

The devolution of Scotland and Wales also offers opportunities for the future development of a service more tailored to the health needs of remote and rural communities in these areas of the UK.

New ways of delivering care out of hours, the ongoing work to define the special nature of rural healthcare, rapid developments in ICT helping to break down distance barriers and the ongoing pressure to move care from secondary into primary care all suggest that the resources will be found to develop rural practice into an even more stimulating and rewarding future.

Summary

- Rural practice has long been bedevilled by its isolation.
- Recent interest and research are beginning to define and celebrate its differences, challenges and successes.
- Increasing devolution in Scotland and Wales has led to greater political attention to issues of rural healthcare.

References

1   Rousseau N (1995) What is rurality? In: J Cox (ed) *Rural General Practice in the UK*. RCGP Occasional Paper No. 71. Royal College of General Practitioners, London, pp. 1–4.

2   Campbell NC, Elliott AM, Sharp L, Cassidy J and Little J (2000) Rural factors and survival from cancer: analysis of Scottish cancer registrations. *British Journal of Cancer*. **82**(11): 1863–6.

3   Baird AG, Donnelly M, Miscampbell N and Wemyss H (2000) Centralisation of cancer services has disadvantages *BMJ*. **320**: 717.

4   Campbell NC, Ritchie LD, Cassidy J and Little J (1999) Systematic review of cancer treatment programmes in remote and rural areas. *British Journal of Cancer*. **80**: 1275–80.

5   Grant J, Ramsay A and Bain J (1997) Medical students and external attachments in community hospitals. *Medical Education*. **31**: 364–8.

6   Lewis R (1996) *Community Hospitals in Scotland: promoting progress*. University of Aberdeen, Aberdeen.

7   Baird AG, Jewell D and Walker JJ (1996) Management of labour in an isolated rural maternity hospital. *BMJ*. **312**: 223–6.

8   Phillimore P and Reading R (1992) A rural disadvantage? Urban-rural health differences in northern England. *Journal of Public Health Medicine*. **14**: 290–9.

9   Cox J (1997) Rural general practice: a personal view of the current key issues. *Health Bulletin*. **55**(5): 309–15.

10   Research into the effect of rurality on the Capitation Formula for Health & Social Services in Northern Ireland, PricewaterhouseCoopers, September 1998.

11   Croft P, Coggon D *et al.* (1992) Osteoarthritis of the hip: an occupational disease in farmers. *BMJ*. **304**: 1269–72.

12   Boulanger S, Deaville J, Randall-Smith J and Wynn-Jones J (1999) *Farm Suicide in Rural Wales: a report of research funded by the Welsh Office*. Institute of Rural Health, Newtown, Powys.

13   Evans A (1999) *Farm Accidents in Rural Areas*. IRH Briefing Paper No. 2. Institute of Rural Health, Newtown, Powys.

14   Baird AG, Gillies JCM *et al.* (1989) Prevalence of antibody indicating Lyme disease in farmers in Wigtownshire. *BMJ*. **299**: 836–7.

15   Gillies JCM (1993) *Mortality in a rural practice*. Abstract in WONCA/SIMG Congress, Nederlands Huisarten Genootschap, p. 116.

16   Baker M, Williams J and Petchey R (1995) GPs in principle but not in practice; a study of vocationally trained doctors not currently working as principals. *BMJ*. **310**: 1301–4.

17   Ross S and Gillies J (1999) Characterics and career intentions of Scottish urban and rural GP registrars. *Health Bulletin*. **57**(1): 44–52.

18   Gillies JCM (1998) Remote and rural practice. *BMJ Classified*. **24 October**.

19   WONCA World Council (1995) *Policy for Training for Rural Practice*. WONCA, Hong Kong.

20   Rousseau N and McColl E (1997) *Equity and Access in Rural Primary Care: an exploratory study in Northumberland and Cumbria, Report No. 83*. Centre for Health Services Research, University of Newcastle upon Tyne.

21   Wootton R (1999) Telemedicine and isolated communities: a UK perspective. *Journal of Telemedicine & Telecare*. **5**(Suppl 2): S27–34.

22 Kunkler IH, Rafferty P, Hill DM, Henry M and Foreman D (1997) Telemedicine proved acceptable in pilot study in Scotland. *BMJ.* **314**: 521

23 Department of Health (2000) *Raising Standards for Patients: new partnerships for out-of-hours care.* Department of Health, London.

24 Marshall L (1997) Associate general practitioners. *Career Focus. BMJ Classified.* **26 July**.

25 Farmer J (1999) Williams Dorothy. Rural information deprivation. *Health Libraries Review.* **16**: 209–12.

26 Cox L and Mungall I (eds) (1998) *Rural Healthcare.* Radcliffe Medical Press, Oxford.

27 Mungall IJ, Wynn Jones J and Deaville J (2001) Rural general practice in the United Kingdom. In: JP Geyman, TE Norris and LG Hart (eds) *Textbook of Rural Medicine.* McGraw-Hill, New York.

28 Department of Environment, Transport and Regions (2000) *A Fair Deal for Rural England: the countryside white paper.* DETR, London.

Recommended additional reading

- Cox J (ed) (1995) *Rural General Practice in the UK.* RCGP Occasional Paper No. 71. RCGP, London.
- Rousseau N, McColl E and Eccles M (1994) *Primary Health Care in Rural Areas: issues of equity and resource management – a literature review.* Centre for Health Services Research, University of Newcastle upon Tyne.

PART 3

Living the future

CHAPTER 13

What doctors want

Isobel Allen

This chapter explores the changing aspirations of today's young doctors, who demand new ways of working and fresh models of professional leadership.

We have heard a lot in the last two or three years about an exodus of doctors. Young doctors are said to be leaving in droves, with reports of 25% dropping out by the time they are 30. But there is little hard evidence that young doctors are leaving the profession in any greater numbers than before and it is likely that the real drop-out rate in the postgraduate years is considerably lower than these dramatic figures suggest.[1] The proportion of qualified doctors who are lost to the profession forever remains very low, some would say surprisingly low.

However, there is plenty of evidence that the aspirations of young doctors are changing. These aspirations and expectations are not being met and young doctors are articulating their dissatisfaction in a variety of ways. They may not be dropping out, but what we appear to be seeing is an increasing tendency to take time off between jobs, not to rush into long-term career choices, to take locum posts, to work in part-time posts, to go abroad and in other ways to drop out of the statistics, which are at the same time becoming increasingly unreliable in measuring the actual activity of the medical workforce.

But nobody should be sanguine about the prospects for the future. Young doctors may not be leaving now, but there are many indications that they are becoming increasingly disillusioned and that it is only their strong sense of vocation and commitment to patients that is preventing them from looking to other areas of work which offer more reasonable conditions and – perhaps most important – allow them the freedom to lead a 'normal life'.[2]

The context

It is important to look at the changing context in which we should examine the question of the morale of young doctors. The profile of the medical profession has been changing rapidly over the past ten years. Women accounted for only 25% of those entering the profession in the 1960s, but the proportion has been rising steadily since then and women have accounted for around 50% of medical graduates for most of the 1990s.[3] In some specialities, for example general practice, well over half of new entrants are women, and that trend looks set to accelerate.[4]

At the same time, there are powerful forces in society which have affected the world of work and employment practices. No longer can anyone expect to work for 40 years in the same place in the same job, and medicine is no exception.[5] Gone are the days when the government had to pass legislation to ensure that doctors would retire at 70. Now there are many indications that early retirement is attractive to many middle-aged doctors, and, perhaps more important, also to younger doctors.

There is also an increasing desire for flexibility within the workforce and this is mirrored in the medical profession. There is a wish for a flexibility which allows part-time or less than full-time working without affecting career prospects – a flexibility which allows doctors to move as consultants or GP principals or to stay put as junior doctors for longer periods than the traditional six months if they want to. There is also increasing evidence that doctors, like others, can become bored and burnt out even in their thirties, especially if they feel that they have no chance of widening their horizons professionally. And this is undoubtedly true of GPs who wish to develop their interest or expertise in another speciality, only to find few opportunities available other than clinical assistant sessions unless they are willing to undergo another lengthy postgraduate training period.

The necessity to find a speciality and stick to it if you want to get on appears to be getting stronger and yet there have always been many doctors who are not certain of which speciality to follow at the end of medical school or even three or four years later. Perhaps it is not surprising that some young doctors are taking their time to make up their minds on a long-term career and yet they must be aware that, in taking their time, they may be missing the boat.

And finally, the profile of the medical profession has changed radically, not only through the great increase in the proportion of women but in other ways. Doctors are becoming far more like their contemporaries outside medicine, with fewer qualifiers coming from medical families, far more coming from state schools and far more with very good A-level results, mainly in science subjects.[3] The motivation of younger doctors has also been changing over the past 20 years, with clear evidence that more recent generations have wanted to study medicine because they were good at science, which raises the question of whether being good at science is necessarily a prerequisite for being a good doctor or even whether good scientists always make good – and happy – doctors.[6]

Causes for disillusionment

What are the causes of the disillusionment? I have carried out a number of studies over the past ten years or so which have identified the most important factors causing problems for young doctors.[3,7,8] Some issues have been tackled in recent years, most particularly the excessively long hours worked by most junior doctors when I conducted the first study of doctors and their careers back in 1986.[7] However, other problems are only now being fully addressed, while others have emerged or have been exacerbated in the past few years.

There are five main areas which cause problems for young doctors. First, the career structure in medicine, which has been described by successive cohorts in my studies as being rigid and inflexible; second, the haphazard nature of careers advice, information and counselling; third, the lack of personal support systems and networks in medicine; fourth, the conditions of work, some of which are simply examples of bad housekeeping by management while others are perhaps more serious and deep-rooted and are illustrated by increasing professional isolation in a culture where territorial boundaries and working practices seem to be inhibiting the development of teamwork and skill mix; fifth, there are increasing indications of stress and disillusionment among young doctors caused by what they feel to be an erosion of their professional values through a managerial culture which they find hostile, intrusive and aggressive. In this chapter, I will explore some of the tensions inherent in this clash of cultures which were illustrated in a recent study examining the views of younger doctors on the core values of medicine.[9]

The career structure in medicine

Doctors from all generations studied in my research have perceived the career structure in medicine as unnecessarily rigid and designed for people who were prepared and able to pursue careers which demanded constant moves in the early years, long hours, full-time working and a very long period of postgraduate training, particularly in the most prestigious special-ities. At the same time, it was thought that those who could operate the system known as patronage made greater progress than others. There seemed little doubt in the minds of most of those interviewed that this system was better-suited to ambitious young men than bright young women.

There is no doubt that there have been a number of changes in recent years which have helped to improve the medical career structure, not least the Calman reforms[10] which have considerably shortened the period of postgraduate training in hospital medicine and have enabled the introduc-tion of much more structured training programmes.

However, in spite of many attempts to introduce more flexible postgrad-uate training opportunities – starting back in the late 1960s and immorta-lised in the PM(79) scheme of blessed memory[11] which facilitated part-time training for senior registrars with strong domestic reasons for wishing to train part time – there is considerable evidence that, in spite of the Calman reforms, there are still difficulties in flexible training, in both hospital medicine and general practice.

In my last study, looking at 1986 qualifiers five years after graduation and comparing them with their 1981 counterparts,[3] there was overwhelming support, among both men and women, for more opportu-nities for flexible training, but only a tiny proportion of doctors had such posts. There is still a strong feeling that less than full-time training is something which should be considered only by those who really have no alternative, both in hospital medicine and general practice. And in spite of the increasing numbers of women entering medicine and the shortage of trainees in certain specialities, not least in general practice, there is still a fear among young doctors that those undertaking less than full-time training are not regarded as 'proper' doctors by their more senior colleagues.

In my study of part-time working in general practice published in 1992, which reported the views of some 1300 GPs who had received vocational training certificates during the 1980s, we found that the vast majority of the women and three-quarters of the men thought that there should be more opportunities for part-time training in general practice.[8] But, again, very few respondents of either sex had done it, mainly because of a lack of available opportunities. There was strong evidence of an unmet demand for such posts.

But it is not only in training posts that young doctors want more flexible working patterns. It is also true among consultants and GP principals. In the study on part-time working in general practice, many of the problems now emerging in the recruitment and retention of GPs were signalled, not least the desire for more part-time opportunities for both men and women as GP principals.[8] There were also problems with partnerships, especially if young doctors had to be geographically mobile, like women who were married to other doctors who were moving around the country in hospital posts. These young doctors were not asking for the earth. One young principal said that she would be helped by her husband getting a consultant post within 30 miles of her practice. Another spoke of the strains on her marriage of living 100 miles away from her husband whom she saw only at weekends. There were undoubtedly problems for young women – and also for young men – about buying into the premises, issues about partnership agreements, difficulties about getting out of partnerships and, not least, problems with financial shares.

There was also clear evidence of older male full-time GP principals wanting to reduce their work commitment in general practice, either to increase other medical work or to pursue other interests, and indications that men wanted to reduce their full-time commitment towards the end of their careers.

There are many other examples of the need for increasing flexibility in the medical profession, which is not noted for speed of change. Perhaps one of the most important is the extent to which young doctors in my most recent cohort study[3] resented being undervalued in the medical hierarchy. The increasingly well-qualified young people entering the medical profession are not as prepared as their predecessors to accept such a hierarchical culture, but at the same time find it difficult to criticise or complain for fear of being branded troublemakers or 'unsound'. The almost obsessive attachment of doctors to their CVs and their references was one of the most striking features for me when I started my research and even in my most recent work[9] I was reminded again of the power of the medical profession in freezing out those who do not conform to structures and practices which might be considered outmoded in other walks of life.

Striking words and expressions have been used by young doctors in my research to describe their lives in their pre-registration year and the years immediately afterwards – being 'treated like clerks' or 'little ants at the bottom of the heap' or 'underdogs' in an atmosphere characterised by 'back stabbing' and 'boot licking'. They felt the training element of their work was being sacrificed for the service element. Perhaps some of these aspects are changing now, but it does seem extraordinary that such highly qualified young people in their mid- and late twenties are being treated in a way which seems designed to undermine their self-esteem and professional status. Many of the young women interviewed had achieved much better grades than the men in their A-levels and yet were saying that they had not thought themselves good enough for hospital medicine. There still appears to be a strong culture within some teaching hospitals that only the 'best' students are fit for hospital medicine, while general practice is all right for the rest. But how do you assess the 'best' students and what are the criteria for a 'good' doctor?

Careers advice, information and counselling

The second theme leads on from this and is concerned with careers advice, information and counselling. All my studies have shown that school careers advice about a medical career is regarded as poor or non-existent in most cases. Although there appears to have been some improvement over the years, it is still thought to be generally ill informed, and many are still discouraged from even contemplating medicine while others, particularly those who are good at science, are encouraged when perhaps they would have been happier as scientists or doing something quite different.[12]

Advice at medical school has been described as not much better and even the latest generation of doctors studied in my research described it as inadequate and not tailored to the personal requirements of individuals. It still seemed to be rather haphazard and offered informally on the job. Again, young doctors were concerned about expressing any doubts or worries about future careers to any member of staff in case this would be regarded as a sign of weakness. There was almost no discussion or advice on important options such as flexible training or part-time career posts, in spite of the fact that so many women were likely to want to work less than full time at some point in their careers. Advice about a career in general practice was regarded as particularly inadequate.

By the time we interviewed the last cohort of doctors four years after registration, only 60% of the men and less than half the women were still in the speciality they had chosen at registration. This not only highlights the danger of making assumptions about career intentions from what people say they are going to do, but it also underlines the inadequacy of much of the careers advice given to medical students and young doctors. Medicine can offer such an enormously wide range of careers under one generic umbrella and yet so many of the young doctors we have interviewed over the years seem to have found it very difficult to find the speciality to suit them. It is probable that some of the disillusionment experienced by young doctors arises because they enter the wrong speciality for the wrong reasons with very little help and advice. And of course, it must never be forgotten that some young doctors are actually in the wrong job. The comments of one young GP were echoed time and again in all the studies: 'I wanted to be a scientist and was misinformed about what it would be like to be a doctor.'

But it is not only in hospital medicine that careers advice in the postgraduate years is rather hit and miss. In the study of GPs, we found considerable criticisms of careers advice and support in general practice, not only from women who found careers advice patchy and limited but also from young men who found little support from more senior doctors. A young GP principal said: 'When one finishes vocational training no attempt is made to find out what one is doing, whether you have a job or not and certainly no assistance given to you to find one. Established GPs care as little about this situation as the consultants, i.e. not at all.' And his views were confirmed by another man: 'The training is haphazard. The advancement is erratic. The overwhelming feeling is that your employer doesn't give a damn. This is very different from industry where people are seen as a valuable resource.'

Lack of personal support systems

The third theme in this chapter is related to the first two – the lack of personal support systems in medicine. There has been a traditional under-development of proper tutorial systems at medical schools, in which discussions on progress may be shared and doubts and fears may be expressed. Things are changing but the system is still patchy and there still seems to be considerable reluctance for medical students to admit doubts which may be seen as a sign of weakness. I have learnt in the course of my research that doctors are never allowed to be 'weak'.

And the lack of personal support systems continues in the postgraduate years. It is difficult to develop proper relationships, either personally or professionally, when you are constantly on the move in your first postgraduate years. But what is depressing is that in many ways the opportunities for developing personal support systems appear to be getting worse rather than better. Unfortunately, this seems to be partly the result of the reduction in junior doctors' hours. At least in the past junior doctors were more likely to be working in a team, with overlap of hours and duties, but now we find increasing evidence of young doctors working on their own, with little support from either their seniors or, perhaps more important, their contemporaries. One doctor in the core values research[9] described himself: 'You don't feel as though you belong. You're this floating nomad in a white coat and stethoscope …'. And a young woman who said, 'I have wept with loneliness' was by no means the only one – male or female – who spoke of acute despair and isolation.

There is also plenty of evidence that general practice can be a very lonely existence with often little support from colleagues and friction within partnerships. Stress levels are high among GPs and recent research has shown correspondingly high levels of anxiety and clinical depression.[13] Professional autonomy is all very well, but it can have a downside.

Conditions of work

The fourth theme is concerned with the conditions of work of young doctors. All through my studies I have recorded the statements made by doctors about the long hours, the on-call system, the constant grind, the intensity of the work and the need to move around the country every six months, particularly in the early postgraduate years. But older doctors have responded to these criticisms by saying that their hours were longer and that they had to work just as hard. What does seem to have changed is not only the intensity of the work – with very ill patients in hospital for a shorter period and increasingly demanding and sophisticated treatments and technology – but also the conditions under which the young doctors are working. There is general agreement that older doctors were looked after much more when they were working those long hours, that their rooms were cleaned, that they had hot meals, a proper bed, clean sheets and were not constantly being bleeped.

But it is not only lack of personal comfort or overwork which contributes towards disillusionment. Increasingly, there is evidence of what can only be called bad housekeeping, which affects not only the work of young doctors but also patient care. Examples abound of poorly maintained equipment, territorial disputes about who does what, lack of co-operation among hospital staff, lack of cleanliness in hospitals and evidence of doctors doing tasks which should be the responsibility of others. Again, in the core values research, discussions were dominated by examples of the inappropriate use of medical skills, which appeared to be grossly inefficient as well as a waste of scarce resources and a major contributory factor in the creation of disillusioned doctors.

Erosion of core values

Finally, I would like to draw on my recent study on the extent to which younger doctors are as committed as older doctors to the core values of the medical profession.[9] These core values were identified as the nine 'ancient virtues distilled over time' at a conference held by leaders of the medical profession at the end of 1994.[14] They include commitment, caring, compassion, integrity, competence, spirit of enquiry, confidentiality, responsibility and advocacy.

In the group discussions held with young doctors under the age of 40, graphic illustrations were given of the factors which were causing disillusionment. Some of these undoubtedly contribute to a climate in which younger doctors might leave the profession. They also give clear indications of where things need to change if they are to stay in medicine, not just under sufferance because it is too difficult to find an alternative career, but where they can fulfil their aspirations and expectations.

How did these young doctors see themselves? They were agreed that they were as committed, if not more committed, to medicine and their patients as their older counterparts. They described themselves as more approachable, more prepared to share information and communicate with patients, give patients time, demystify the medical profession and to acknowledge to patients that they were not divine. They were more prepared to work in teams, to recognise the need for management and audit and all kinds of other things that they thought some of their older colleagues were a little suspicious of.

But there were indications that they felt a constant erosion of their professional autonomy. Many of these young doctors had entered the medical profession with a sense of vocation, but had implicitly balanced the demands of a total commitment to their patients and to medicine with the benefits of the autonomy which went with their professional training and status. There was evidence in all the groups that this trade-off between commitment and autonomy was being affected by pressures from management, patients and society in general.

The animosity expressed towards management by most of these young doctors was striking. There was overwhelming agreement that management did not share their value systems. Most doctors stressed their desire to retain their clinical autonomy, to maintain close contact with their patients and to provide a service which was dictated by the needs of patients and not by the demands of managers and administrators. They felt that their clinical autonomy and professional integrity were being continually challenged and this was an important contributory factor to the increased stress they felt themselves to be under.

GPs and hospital doctors alike were concerned about the extent to which their practice was being ordered by factors outside their control. There were many indications that they could cope with the increasing expectations of patients, as long as these were not dominated by charter requirements and unrealistic demands. GPs in particular were unhappy about being treated as a 'pizza parlour' which could be called upon to supply a service at any time of the day and night.

These doctors saw themselves very clearly as the patient's advocate and resented implications that nurses wished to supplant them in this role. But although they identified themselves as the individual patient's advocate, most wished to take part in discussions on rationing and prioritisation, the terms of which they felt were often being dictated by managers and administrators. They felt they had a clear contribution to make to any debate on the wider needs of society while retaining their role as the patient's advocate.

Discussion of the core value of 'spirit of enquiry' was sadly lacking in these groups. The sheer grind of keeping their heads above water appeared to have put paid to any pursuit of that among these doctors, many of whom had started their careers as brilliant young scientists.

But permeating all the discussions was the fact that these young doctors saw the need for change in the future. They felt that the medical profession should take a leadership role, based not on traditional power and mystique but on clinical knowledge, sound judgement and commitment to the core values of medicine. Otherwise, they would find themselves sidelined and treated as 'technical monkeys' by a management culture which did not share their values but put increased throughput and numbers above competence, care and compassion. It is to be hoped that the leaders of the medical profession – and the government – listen very carefully to what younger doctors are saying, because otherwise there is a grave danger that more of them will begin to speak with their feet.

Summary

- Although not leaving the profession, many young doctors are disillusioned.
- The medical career structure is rigid and inflexible.
- Both personal and professional support systems for doctors are poor.
- Many doctors feel stressed and isolated.
- Many also feel a constant erosion of their professional autonomy.
- In the future, doctors must take a lead based on clinical skill and medical core values.

References

1   Richards P, McManus C and Allen I (1997) British doctors are not disappearing. *BMJ*. **314**: 1567–8.
2   Richards T (1997) Disillusioned doctors. *BMJ*. **314**: 1705–6.

3   Allen I (1994) *Doctors and their Careers: a new generation.* Policy Studies Institute, London.

4   Department of Health (1997) *Statistics for General Medical Practitioners in England: 1986–1996.* Department of Health, London.

5   Allen I (1996) Career preferences of doctors. *BMJ.* **313**: 2.

6   Allen I, Brown P and Hughes P (eds) (1997) *Choosing Tomorrow's Doctors.* Policy Studies Institute, London.

7   Allen I (1988) *Doctors and their Careers.* Policy Studies Institute, London.

8   Allen I (1992) *Part-time Working in General Practice.* Policy Studies Institute, London.

9   Allen I (1997) *Committed but Critical: an examination of young doctors' views of their core values.* BMA, London.

10   Department of Health (1993) *Hospital Doctors: training for the future. The Report of the Working Group on Specialist Medical Training (The Calman Report).* Department of Health, London.

11   Department of Health and Social Security (1979) *Opportunities for Part-time Training in the NHS for Doctors and Dentists with Part-time Commitments, Disability or Ill-health.* PM(79)3. Department of Health and Social Security, London.

12   Carnall D (1997) Career guidance for doctors. *BMJ.* **315**: 6.

13   Chambers R, quoted by Stuttaford T (1997) in *The Times*, **8 August**.

14   British Medical Association (1995) *Core Values for the Medical Profession in the 21st Century: conference report.* BMA, London.

CHAPTER 14

What patients expect

Marianne Rigge

This chapter describes the future from the patients' point of view. More information for patients and greater patient involvement in planning and delivering services are envisaged, as well as better collaboration amongst services.

Looking back

When asked to look into the future, it is sometimes salutary to start by looking back to the past and to what you yourself once thought and said about the future you now find yourself in. More often than not, you find that the problems of the past are still with us. Perhaps this is because human nature does not change much, even though industrial, economic or information technology revolutions may make it seem as though we are on the brink of a brave or frightening new world. *Plus ça change, plus c'est la même chose.*

Back in the 1980s, the then Conservative government announced that it was to conduct a comprehensive review of primary healthcare services in the NHS.[1] Rereading the College of Health's response to this Green Paper provoked a profound sense of *déjà vu*.

> Raising the quality of primary care may lie, not so much in giving extra rewards to those who are already providing high quality services, as in finding ways of discouraging poor practice ... Unfortunately, as successive reports have shown, most notably the 1981 Acheson Report, it is the very people who are already most socially disadvantaged, and most in need of high quality primary health care, because of their relatively high levels of

mortality and morbidity, who are most likely to be on the receiving end of an unacceptably low standard of care.[2]

Yet here we are, at the beginning of the new millennium and the figures for mortality and morbidity amongst the most disadvantaged are still much the same. Considerable numbers of single-handed GPs are still practising from lock-up premises in the inner cities. There have been widespread hospital and bed closures. Trolley waits are an unpleasant new phenomenon and acute beds are being blocked by elderly medical patients who should probably not be in them in the first place. The promised 'care in the community' has not been delivered in what was supposed to be a system of 'seamless' care. For all too many patients and their carers, it seems that less care is available.

How does that rather depressing picture fit into the exciting world that is opening up through advances in information and medical technology, let alone all the rhetoric about empowering consumers, informed choice and evidence-based medicine?

What patients think

In recent years the College of Health carried out four studies of patients' priorities for primary healthcare in the North Western region and two of the Thames regions.[3–6] Besides asking people about the services they currently receive, we posed a range of alternative scenarios for the future, including polyclinics and minor injuries clinics alongside Accident and Emergency departments. Cynicism prevailed.

On the idea of many more consultants doing outreach clinics in GP practices, one patient said:

> You must be joking if you're talking about a consultant coming to these surgeries. You don't even see one if you go to the main hospital. I've been there and all you ever see is their understudies.

On the idea of polyclinics:

> It's an economic fact if you keep it all on one site, a big hospital with more services, that's the most cost-effective way of doing it. If they start setting up these polywhatsits, you know what will happen, they'll close down the hospitals and then where will you be if you haven't got a good GP?

Overwhelmingly, what patients valued most was a good and continuing relationship with a caring GP, backed up by a decent local hospital service and specialist care when they needed it. What the majority of patients also wanted was to be able to get an appointment with their own GP with a minimum of delay and to have a consultation in which they felt they were listened to and able to ask questions. The strength of feeling on this was much greater than on any of the issues which currently preoccupy health service planners, professionals and managers.

Patientville 2003

So where do we go from here? I have a vision of 'Patientville' in the year 2003 which has been articulated elsewhere insofar as it applies to health authorities and trusts. This is what it looks like from the primary healthcare point of view.

All the district's GPs and their teams practise from well-equipped family health centres which co-operate with one another to provide 24-hour emergency cover with several strategically placed out-of-hours walk-in centres, complete with community pharmacies. These are supplemented by GP and nurse-led telephone information and advice services for patients who are unsure whether they should go to the Accident and Emergency department or whether they can safely treat themselves until they can see their own doctor.

Much effort has gone into ensuring that patients can get easy access to a wide range of information about medical and health topics using several different media. There is, for example, a patient library which includes books, leaflets, tapes and videos. Every patient is given a directory of the 500 Healthline tapes which they can listen to on the phone in the privacy of their own home 24 hours a day, any day of the year on the freephone Health Information Service on 0800 665544. The family health centres also hold factsheets based on the Healthline scripts and translated, where appropriate, into languages to suit the local community. These can be accessed via a touchscreen in the waiting area and patients can print them out if they wish.

One innovation, which has proved popular with GPs as well as patients, is a series of leaflets on common operations and illnesses and their treatment called 'Questions to ask the doctor'. From the patients' point of view, this has been found to make it much easier for them to articulate questions they might otherwise have felt nervous or embarrassed talking about. For the GPs, there is comfort in knowing they have evidence-based answers at their fingertips, without having to resort to textbooks, journals or guidelines.

Studies have shown that not only do patients greatly welcome the ease of access to information and the feeling of control it gives them, but it can also substantially reduce inappropriate demands on the healthcare team:

> A seriously brilliant service! It gave me information I doubt I would have thought to ask the GP for. (Patient)

> Promote it. Using the information I was given, I realised I didn't need to bother the doctor. (Patient)

The family health centres live up to their name in other ways too. Everyone is welcome and their varying needs are catered for. For a start, there is a strong emphasis on keeping healthy.

In Patientville, the GPs are as likely to write out prescriptions for exercise as for drugs and to refer their patients on to nurse practitioners, physiotherapists, stress counsellors or complementary therapists as to hospital specialists. The family health centres offer a wide range of exercise and relaxation facilities, diet clubs, non-judgemental Quit Smoking and Sensible Drinking sessions and encouragement is given to local self-help and community groups to hold meetings on the premises.

Information technology

Information technology has been harnessed in a variety of ways to ensure that care across the boundaries of general practice, hospital, community and social services is thoroughly co-ordinated.

The use of smart cards was quickly abandoned after patients complained that it was offensive for their details to be available to health professionals but not to them. Instead, patients are encouraged to hold a paper version of their own records and to participate actively in drawing up care plans. They are routinely given printed information about any diagnostic tests or operative procedures at the time of referral and are encouraged to tape record consultations if they wish. The take-up rates for immunisation and screening programmes have improved dramatically since the introduction of patient-held records, as patients can see at a glance whether they have missed out on something to which they are entitled. An added benefit for healthcare professionals with whom patients choose to share their records is that they are able to see what other forms of treatment patients are having, for example from complementary therapists or with over-the-counter medications or herbal remedies. These, after all, are not without side effects.

Missed appointment rates have reduced considerably since GPs have had online access to the outpatients department at the district general hospital. They can make appointments while their patients are still with them. This has been further enhanced by the booked admission systems now available to hospital consultants and automatically reported back to GPs.

Patients' involvement in quality assurance

The Patientville GP consortium holds regular meetings with all the clinical directorates from the district general hospital and community health services to agree patient-centred referral and discharge protocols. There are also clearly agreed protocols about what diagnostic tests should be ordered, by whom and at what stage, as well as how, when and by whom the results should be communicated to patients. Although waiting times have been considerably reduced, there is a strong awareness of the need to guide patients towards sources of information, help and advice. This enables them to cope with their illness and get as fit as possible if they do have to wait more than a few weeks for admission. The help includes physiotherapy and occupational therapy, aids and adaptations to the home through social services, welfare and other benefits and referral to self-help groups.

All these protocols, along with patient versions of all the clinical guidelines currently in use, are freely available to patients.

Patients also have access to the anonymised results of clinical audit and research projects. Since the dismantling of the internal market, trusts have become much more open to the idea of cross-boundary and cross-district audit. As a result there is a much less defensive attitude on the part of clinicians to sharing the results. The greater numbers involved make it less likely that individual clinicians' identities can be guessed.

Not only are patients and carers involved in the planning, development, implementation, monitoring and evaluation of guidelines and audit protocols, they are also positively encouraged to feed back information about how they have been treated in other parts of the healthcare system. It is recognised that patients who are well informed about good practice are much more likely to report back in a positive and constructive way on whether or not guidelines have been followed.

Consumer audits are another method of ensuring that services remain patient focused. In-depth interviews with patients and carers, focus groups and observation with the help of checklists all form part of the quality assurance methodology. Particular attention is paid to gathering information about patients' views of outcomes. It is recognised that they are the ultimate arbiters of whether an outcome has been successful. This change in practice followed the realisation that people who turn to general practice for help rarely present with a single 'evidence-based illness' that can be neatly categorised according to the results of a randomised controlled trial. Such trials, almost by definition, exclude the vast majority of practice populations whose age, sex or co-morbidities might 'spoil the science'!

For much the same reason, both GPs and patients have much more information than was available in the past about consultants and their special interests and about centres of expertise. As a result patients with straightforward needs for day or elective surgery might opt for the shortest waiting list. Others, with more complicated or serious problems, can ask to be referred to the specialist and team best suited to them.

Conclusion

Most of the patient-centred practices imagined in Patientville are not, in fact, imaginary at all. They are part of everyday general practice somewhere in the UK already. The future may not be the uncharted foreign country we fear but rather a much better thought through and signposted version of the landscape we already know.

Summary

- In spite of change, many problems endure.
- Above all, patients want a good and continuing relationship with a caring GP.
- Patients will have much better access to information.
- Professionals will need to engage with patients in planning services and ensuring their quality.
- Much of what is imagined for the future already exists somewhere in the UK.

References

1   Secretaries of State for Social Services, Wales, Northern Ireland and Scotland (1986) *Primary Health Care. An Agenda for Discussion.* Cmnd 9771. HMSO, London.

2   East London and the City Health Authority (1998) *Health in the East End. Annual Public Health Report 1997/98.* East London and the City Health Authority, London.

3   College of Health (1994) *Patients' Priorities for Primary Medical Care in the North Western Region.* College of Health, London.

4   College of Health (1996) *Patients' Priorities for Primary Health Care in Rainham*

and Thamesview (Report for Barking and Havering FHSA). College of Health, London.

5   College of Health (1996) *Patients' Priorities for Primary Medical Care in Bexley and Greenwich.* College of Health, London.

6   Rigge M (1997) Keeping the customer satisfied. *Health Service Journal.* **30 October**: 24–7.

CHAPTER 15

Regaining control

Jamie Harrison

Why, Hal, 'tis my vocation, Hal; 'tis no sin for a man to labour in his vocation.
Henry IV, part I

This chapter examines how general practitioners and practices respond to change and uncertainty. Coping mechanisms, with five strategies, are suggested.

Uncertainty in general practice

Clinical

All general practitioners have to live with uncertainty in their clinical practice. It is the price they pay for being a family doctor, distanced from the local hospital, where inpatient observation can provide safety and certainty. In the community outside, the chasm between home and hospital cannot be measured in miles. Psychologically and emotionally, the feeling of distance is all-pervasive. The questions come thick and fast. Should I revisit the sick patient, refer or admit? How do I cope with not knowing what is round the corner? Is my medical defence subscription up to date?

For young general practitioners, this sense of 'distance' can be emotionally difficult. Their training, however, reminds them that:

- most presenting symptoms are expressions of benign conditions
- dangerous illnesses are rare
- the vast majority of patients get better without medical intervention

- catastrophes do occur, but sensible vigilance and good systems of communication minimise their frequency
- when things go wrong, it is usually as a result of a series of mistakes or errors, each of which on its own would not have led to the disaster.

General practitioners must therefore learn to develop strategies that enable them to handle clinical uncertainty effectively.

Organisational

Latterly any difficulty in managing clinical uncertainty has been compounded by a series of changes, both in society at large and in the organisation of the health service itself, by:

- a government wanting to raise standards and to hold down healthcare costs
- a society developing its consumerist edge, demanding accountability in services provided and high quality of care across the board
- a thriving pharmaceutical and medical research sector, flush with new products, technologies and techniques, bombarding the medical profession with the latest possibilities
- a powerful and pervasive media, communicating medical knowledge and wisdom to all
- ever-increasing medical litigation
- an accelerating rate of change itself.

General practitioners then have to contend with uncertainty both in their clinical practice and in the environment in which they work. One without the other would be stressful. The two combined are a potent cause of anxiety.

Maladaptive responses to change and uncertainty

Ideally, the environment in which general practitioners work should enable them to realise their full potential. This would bring immense benefit not only to themselves but also to patient care and the organisation.[1] Unfortunately, the way in which some practices are organised and managed puts pressure and stress on to individuals, preventing such benefits accruing to themselves or to their patients.

These practices lack good people skills, dynamic strategic planning or a well-developed structure for training and education. Individuals are left to 'get on with it'. The work itself is more than enough. The lack of a coherent overview allied to a reactive pattern of response to change and pressure leaves the practice struggling. In these circumstances, defensive routines develop, locking practices and practitioners in 'survival mode', where any change is a threat and no change best of all.[2]

A role play by some North London GP tutors[3] highlighted the difficulties of such a family doctor under pressure. Simple organisational changes were mountains to climb. Cut off from peers and suspicious of offers of help from the local health authority, the doctor put up barriers to external support and retrenched further into his shell. He felt overwhelmed by paperwork and patient demand.

Where defence becomes the only option, the working day is reduced to the performance of routine tasks. Reaching the end of the day unscathed is the target. There is then:

- no vision of what the work is truly about
- no understanding of whether the effort is successful
- no view of what might be achieved in the longer term.

Such a state leads to passivity in the face of challenge and a resigned acceptance of change, if only to limit the damage which the change threatens. Risk of burnout is increased and there is a longing for escape. Early retirement, part-time working or even a job change may beckon, but the well-defended GP is unable to see the possibilities such a change might offer.

Defensive responses to stress

The British psychotherapist Robert Hale has spent time counselling medical practitioners in need of help. He has identified a range of psychological defences used by doctors in response to work-related stress. He categorised four strategies such doctors use for their own survival.

Denial

We are all familiar with the concept of denial, where we reject the notion of anxiety or tension within ourselves. Whatever the problem confronting us, we believe we can cope and maintain our professional performance. Hale likens this to riding a tiger, for 'He who rides the tiger dare not dismount.' Once off the tiger, we must face our failures and fears, so better to keep riding! He notes that those who reduce their hours of work can experience more feelings of stress, 'perhaps because if you stop you have to face all the pain'.[4] One wonders whether this might explain why so many more female (presumed often less than full-time) general practitioners contact stress helplines than their male counterparts.[5] Or perhaps the women are just more in touch with their feelings and willing to seek guidance. There may be a message here for all.

Altruism

Altruism is cited as an unexpected defence mechanism, but it can protect doctors from conflict and anxiety. It can also be dangerous, as doctors may feel an overwhelming call to be there and to care for patients, whatever the cost.[6] Yet, as Isobel Allen found, altruism may be the only thing that keeps some young doctors in medicine.[7] Properly balanced, altruism can give shape and meaning to a professional life, but it cannot compensate for significant stress for long.

Intellectualising

Many doctors seek to escape from the demands of patients by intellectualising, or medicalising, their work. The patient is no longer a person, but a knee, a liver or a spleen. In this way, the demand for care by someone is replaced by the need to deal with something.

A similar mechanism may be at work with the tendency to demonise and stereotype managers and politicians. By reducing them to caricature, it is easier to distance oneself from the need to engage with them as people. For to admit that your perceived opponents are trying their best, and to try to see things from their perspective, changes the way we see the world.

Acting out

One further defence mechanism is that of acting out. Here, the doctor tries to avoid that which is painful by an action which may itself be harmful.[8] Some doctors drink too much. Others self-medicate or commit suicide. Work itself can become a way out, by frenetic overwork, where medical over-activity may have its roots in the need actually to *do* something, rather than to wait patiently in the wings.

Regaining control

There are few more fearful experiences than feeling that control over one's own destiny is slipping away, either personally or professionally. Reclaiming a sense of direction becomes an imperative. Five strategies are proposed for regaining control of a GP career (Box 15.1). Each of these strategies has benefits, not only for general practitioners who are struggling but also for general practitioners in general.

Box 15.1 Five strategies for regaining control

- Value a sense of vocation.
- Discover your career anchor.
- Develop a portfolio career.
- Regain professional control.
- Innovate and be better managed.

Valuing a sense of vocation

When pressures come, it is easier to cope when there is a pre-existing sense of the rightness of doing the job. An appreciation and ownership of the historic core values of the profession leads to greater personal fulfilment:

> I am still a doctor, destined for more uncertain times, unmanageable days, undeserved rewards, and the inexhaustible opportunity to touch the lives of those I treat. And to change their lives as they have changed mine. Our work bears the stamp of a centuries-old tradition and is carried forward by each new class of physicians.[9]

In a post-modern world, where feelings and perceptions are thought to have a particular role, having a sense of vocation or calling to medicine may be not only the best reason for being a doctor, but also the force that sustains doctors at times of stress. Awareness of the traditions of the medical profession gives shape and coherence to medical practice. Within the role or 'character' of a doctor, the individual finds meaning and that ability to withstand the pressures which come from change.[6,10]

A sense of vocation has been derided by some[11] but historically general practitioners have maintained their social and psychological equilibrium by seeing themselves as part of a bigger picture, as those set apart, with others, to serve the community. There are benefits in valuing this notion which is enshrined in the very wording of general practitioner training – vocational training for general practice. The late Clare Vaughan pointed this out in her request for a new experience of such a vocation:

How can the job be redefined to engage a new sense of vocation while retaining elements of the work that continue to satisfy? Our challenge is to find teaching, vocational training, and lifelong personal and professional development.[12]

Discovering your career anchor

The career anchor is that self-understanding individuals develop in relation to what they do well.[13] This awareness, of talents, motives and attitudes, based on actual experience, provides a stabilising 'anchor' to maintain a career. Accurately defined, the career anchor can help in planning future career and life options.

Edgar Schein has studied career anchors for management graduates from the Massachusetts Institute of Technology (MIT). Typical career anchors for these graduates were:

- technical competence
- managerial competence
- security
- autonomy.

Schein fleshed out his ideas as follows:

> For example, one graduate using a technical competence anchor was still, in mid-career, only concerned with technical tasks. He refused to become involved in aspects of sales or general management even though he was now a director and part owner of the firm in which he worked. Another graduate, using managerial competence as an anchor, left one firm although his bosses were quite pleased with his performance. But he considered that he only actually worked two hours a day, and he was not satisfied with that.[14]

Schein makes the point that in grasping the concept of career anchors, we are better able to respond to early-, mid- and late-career crises. For general practitioners, the four anchors exhibited by the MIT graduates have relevance.

- Some pride themselves on *technical competence*, whether in consulting, computers, minor surgery, joint manipulation or diagnosis. Medical techniques are all that really matter.
- For others, the opportunity to *manage* has proved rewarding and motivating, with some hailing the opportunity to manage fundholding

activities as the salvation of their mid-career crisis. Commissioning may do the same.

- Job and personal *security* rank high for those who value safe and predictable ways of living; historically, general practitioners have had a secure income and permanent contract with the NHS.
- *Autonomy* may be limited by external forces, which may explain why some doctors appear so irritated by new contractual arrangements. Traditionally, general practitioners have enjoyed a significant degree of autonomy in the way they organise their work.

The danger of an unfulfilled career anchor was shown by Schein's example of the MIT graduate who only valued his two hours a day of 'real work'. He left to find another job which would better satisfy his particular talents and motivation.

Recent emphasis on the doctor as manager has made some general practitioners ask what is central to being a GP. Is it personal patient contact on a daily basis that makes you a 'proper doctor'? Or are general practitioners those doctors who manifest the core values of general practice – those with an ethos arising out of past experience of vocational training, the consultation and being a patient advocate – whether they continue to see patients or not?

Those who no longer have direct patient contact might therefore still satisfy a career anchor defined as 'doing the work of a general practitioner'. Whether such a position can be sustained after a prolonged absence from the consulting room is a moot question.

Developing a portfolio career

Portfolio living

Charles Handy has described how managers, in particular, develop their professional capabilities by concentrating on particular aspects of their work before moving on to something else. Handy himself produced an annual schedule with specific time allocated to particular activities, for example writing, teaching, travel and recreation.

Such 'portfolio living' forces people 'to think in terms of a circle, something like a pie-chart, with different segments marked off for different occupations, each coloured for kind and degree of hoped-for remuneration'. The chart will be constantly changing, not only over the years of one's life but from week to week, even day to day. This deliberate cultivation of multiple expertises characterises the portfolio career, a notion which already excites:

> The best of the portfolio careerists will want challenge and a
> chance to develop in their professional fields, as well as money,
> and they will move to wherever they can find these opportu-
> nities.[15]

For many general practitioners, the traditional career no longer meets their
needs or wishes.[16] Indeed, for generations general practitioners have
involved themselves in activities outside core general practice, such as
occupational medicine, clinical assistantships, teaching, audit and medical
politics. In the future this 'extracurricular' involvement is likely to be more
prominent in doctors' careers, with 'serial' movement from one activity to
another to develop different capabilities. Some doctors will ultimately move
to different careers in management or research, as their portfolio career
develops.

> Doctors with portfolio careers avoid the expectation that their job
> will continue the same for 30 years, have a richer professional
> life, and prevent burnout. A varied portfolio would accommodate
> family life and maternity and paternity leaves and prepare for an
> active retirement.[17]

Not all professional activities will receive payment in money; there will be
other kinds of (unpaid) reward – love, creative satisfaction, power or joy.
Yet, for all its fluidity, flexibility and professional challenge, the portfolio
career will not be universally attractive:

> The portfolio life will not be to everyone's taste. It maximizes
> freedom at the expense of security, an ancient trade-off.[15]

With freedom comes the risk of over-commitment and exhaustion, as
multiple part-time jobs virtually always add up to more than one full-time
job. In addition, a crisis in one activity can place undue pressure on all the
others.

Flexible training and part-time working

Allied to the concept of portfolio living is the adoption of new flexibilities in
work patterns. Part-time training[18] and working arrangements allow
greater freedom to pursue personal goals. Career breaks, the option to
change working hours and job-sharing opportunities merely reflect what is
normal in the world outside medicine. Both established principals and newly
trained general practitioners suggest that six to seven surgeries per week is
the ideal workload, creating space for other medical and social interests.[19]

Helen Gibson has argued that working part time brings more humanity and a greater understanding of patients and the real world.[20] For her, the traditional ethos of medicine values 'single-minded commitment, continuity of care, and success linked to age'. As a result, part-time workers are under-valued, perceived as being uncommitted and unwilling to put in the neces-sary career effort. Indeed, there are other flaws in the traditional viewpoint she highlights. As one vocational registrar noted recently, 'Doctors offered everything on the basis that patients wouldn't ask too much.'[21] The myth of constant availability can only be sustained when the doctor knows that the patients will not act as if it were true. Most doctors do not want to work long hours. They desire a decent family life and leisure time.[22] As one male registrar recently put it:

> The attraction that general practice held for me was not a medical attraction. It was the attraction of being able to run your own business. Be settled in one area. Have a family. Have a dog. All that sort of thing.[23]

In addition, more time spent on other, non-medical activities can make doctors more humane, with a wider view on life,[24] and can reduce the risk of burnout.[25]

Out-of-hours co-operatives have enabled increasing numbers of doctors to enjoy their lives away from the practice. The option for more general practi-tioners to be salaried employees holds out the possibility of a new freedom for others.[26] This new menu of partnership and salaried opportunities, both full-time and part-time, will be attractive to many, as long as the old dangers of exploitation and poor salaries are avoided.[27] Improved career guidance, with ongoing career advice and support, will also help.[28]

Regaining professional control

Regaining professional control touches on issues of quality and account-ability. In an increasingly aware consumerist society, professions can no longer afford to shield themselves behind professional secrecy. To sustain proper accountability, mechanisms for assuring the quality of care need to be transparent through proper regulation and clinical audit.

Demonstrable adherence to evidence-based guidelines would reassure patients, particularly if they (or their representatives) had been involved in constructing the guidelines in the first place. Failure to satisfy the public on issues of quality hastens the imposition of an external monitoring authority similar to OFSTED, the educational inspectorate for teachers and schools. Will this be the role of the Health Improvement Commission cited in the White Paper *The New NHS*?[29]

This issue poses a real challenge, which is being met at least in part by the new General Medical Council (GMC) performance procedures. But much more will be needed and the profession needs to take the initiative, thereby regaining control.

A survey commissioned by the British Medical Association in 1992 showed that nearly two-thirds of British general practitioners believed that initial competence (on entering the profession) would not be enough to sustain a career. Yet little has been done to implement a programme of systematic reappraisal.[30]

Innovation and better management

Effective innovation requires the willingness to take risks, an openness to new ideas, the capability to reflect critically and the ability to act strategically as developments occur. One of these attributes, without the others to balance it, may lead to disaster.

Innovation has occurred since 1990 in the wider use of surgery premises (for example, to house visiting therapists and for minor surgery), delegation to nurses and managers, the development of the nurse practitioner role and the harnessing of information technology. Practices and practitioners have recently set the pace in terms of organisational change, with the creation of purchaser and provider networks of fundholders and commissioning groups (Chapter 2). The opening up of NHS regulations since 1996 has further driven this process forward.

However, not all practices are at the forefront of change, nor would they wish to be. Yet in the face of change, organisations in any field eventually take on the appearance and approach of those around them.[31] This drive to conformity can result from external pressure, for example government, but wise imitation and the beneficial impact of managers play their part. The problems facing one GP practice will be broadly similar to those facing its neighbours. The most innovative practices set the pace and stimulate new organisational patterns, but also make mistakes, from which all can learn lessons. By sharing good ideas and ways of working, healthy organisations develop, imitating each other. Indeed, the best-attended GP postgraduate meetings in 1991 were those devoted to understanding how to cope with the new contractual changes, through hearing the stories of colleagues. This occurred despite the attempt of the government of the day to introduce competition between practices.

When practices experience the benefit of being managed effectively, a process of organisational development occurs. Tasks are delegated appropriately, teamworking is enhanced and improved systems evolve. Clinicians are freed to spend more time on patient care. Better management has developed as:

- managers from outside the health service have joined practices, particularly to relieve the administrative pressures on doctors
- doctors and senior receptionists have themselves taken on more formal managerial roles, often guided and directed by professionally trained managers
- general practitioners have begun to study for degrees in business administration (MBAs)
- doctors have increasingly seen management as a legitimate part of general practice.

Managers bring personal and organisational values with them.[32] Their expertise has made practices more like business organisations and helped them to cope with the continuing pressure of further change.

Conclusion

This chapter has reflected on general practitioners under pressure and on responses to change and uncertainty at work. Five strategies, which focus on reclaiming both personal and professional control, have been highlighted.

Yet all general practitioners face questions about how to increase medical effectiveness while remaining fulfilled and happy in their work. This applies whether or not feelings of stress have become intrusive. Doctors know the value of positive interventions as a way of developing healthy bodies. Time spent on building and sustaining healthy careers would also be worthwhile.

Summary

- All general practitioners live with medical uncertainty.
- Poor organisation can lead to sterile defensive routines.
- Stress at work produces a range of unhelpful responses.
- A sense of vocation provides meaning and purpose for life and work.
- Discovering your career anchor helps to ground you at work.
- Portfolio careers can provide fun and flexibility.
- Part-time working suits many doctors.
- Doctors are beginning to take back control over their destinies.
- GP practices benefit from professional management and imitate each other over time.

References

1 Argyris C (1957) *Personality and Organization*. Harper and Row, New York.
2 Argyris C (1985) *Strategy, Change and Defensive Routines*. Pitman, London.
3 Enacted at the 1996 National GP Tutors' Conference.
4 Hale R (1997) How patients make their doctors ill. In: I Allen, P Brown and P Hughes (eds) *Choosing Tomorrow's Doctors*. Policy Studies Institute, London.
5 Bogle I (1997) Proceedings of the Towards Healthier Doctors Conference. RCGP, 12 November, London.
6 Harrison J and Innes R (1997) *Medical Vocation and Generation X*. Grove Books, Cambridge.
7 Allen I (1997) *Committed but Critical: an examination of young doctors' views of their core values*. BMA, London.
8 Bennet G (1987) *The Wound and the Doctor: healing, technology and power in modern medicine*. Secker and Warburg, London.
9 Loxterkamp D (1996) Hearing voices. How should doctors respond to their calling? *NEJM*. **335**: 1991–3.
10 MacIntyre A (1981) *After Virtue*. Duckworth, London.
11 Harrison J (1996) Is this what we really want? *BMJ*. **313**: 1643.
12 Vaughan C (1995) Career choices for generation X. Young doctors want flexible career paths, not long term commitments. *BMJ*. **311**: 525–6.
13 Schein EH (1993) *Career Anchors: discovering your real values*. Pfeiffer, San Francisco.
14 Pugh DS and Hickson DJ (1996) Edgar H. Schein. In: *Writers on Organizations*. Penguin, London.
15 Handy C (1996) *Beyond Certainty*. Arrow Business Books, London.
16 Crawley H (1996) Building a career portfolio in general practice. *BMJ Classified*. **2 November**.
17 Gray C (1996) Portfolio careers. *BMJ Classified*. **7 September**.
18 Sinha A and Cook A (1997) What do medical students think of flexible training? *BMJ Classified*. **6 December**.
19 Salmon EL (1997) *A Professional Development Year in General Practice. Final Report of the First Two Years of the Vocationally Trained Associate Scheme in Lambeth, Southwark and Lewisham*. South London Organization of Vocational Training Schemes, London.
20 Gibson H (1997) Are part time doctors better doctors? *BMJ Classified*. **11 October**.
21 Vaughan C and Higgs R (1995) Doctors and commitment. Nice work – shame about the job. *BMJ*. **311**: 1654–5.
22 Charlton BG (1993) Holistic medicine or the humane doctor. *British Journal of General Practice*. **43**: 475–7.
23 Petchey R, Williams J and Baker M (1997) 'Ending up a GP': a qualitative study of junior doctors' perceptions of general practice as a career. *Family Practice*. **14**: 194–8.

24   British Medical Association (1995) *Core Values for the Medical Profession in the 21st century.* BMA, London.

25   Kirwan M and Armstrong D (1995) Investigation of burnout in a sample of British general practitioners. *British Journal of General Practice.* **45**: 259–60.

26   National Health Service Executive (1997) *Salaried Doctor's Scheme.* FHSL (97) 46. NHSE, Leeds.

27   Heath I and Amiel S (1997) Safeguards are needed for new proposals for primary care. *BMJ.* **314**: 149.

28   Hutton-Taylor S (1996) Do it yourself career guidance. *BMJ Classified.* **10 August**.

29   Secretary of State for Health (1997) *The New NHS: modern dependable.* HMSO, London.

30   Electoral Reform Ballot Services (1992) *Your Choices for the Future. A Survey of GP Opinion.* General Medical Services Committee, London.

31   Di Maggio PJ and Powell WW (1983) The iron cage revisited: institutional isomorphism and collective rationality in organizational fields. *American Sociological Review.* **48**: 147–60.

32   Shields P (1997) Sense of values. *Human Resources in the NHS.* **17**: 4.

CHAPTER 16

GP tomorrow

Tim van Zwanenberg

Happy the man, and happy he alone;
He, who can call today his own:
He who, secure within, can say,
Tomorrow do thy worst, for I have lived today.
The Odes of Horace (trans. Dryden)

This chapter anticipates what will be required in the future and describes how general practitioners will need to be adept in a variety of skills – not least coping with unending change.

What can we expect?

General practitioners and those involved in primary care more widely will continue to have a critical role in the NHS of the future, not only as organisers and providers of an increasing range and quality of services but also as gatekeepers to and commissioners of hospital-based care.

Change, which has been so evident over the last few years, will go on and may be more radical than presently imagined. The new primary care trusts and care trusts, particularly those arising from mergers of primary care groups, herald the possibility of much larger primary care organisations and the demise of the practice partnership as we know it. Personal Medical Services projects are exploring different ways of organising primary care, and a new quality-based contract for both General and Personal Medical Services is expected. And *NHS Direct* is set to become the out-of-hours front door of primary care.

While many general practitioners may continue as self-employed, independent contractors, a significant and growing proportion will become salaried employees in these larger primary care trusts. There may be different models in rural areas and in conurbations. The performance management of primary care trusts by the new strategic health authorities will develop, as the trusts take on the responsibility for improving the health of the community; securing the provision of services – primary, secondary and community services; and integrating health and social care.[1] Administering the national GP contract will no longer be the main role of the primary care authority, as it was for Family Health Service Authorities only a few years ago, and increasingly, general practitioners, on behalf of their primary care trust, will be expected to assure the quality of care provided by their colleagues through clinical governance.

From the formation of group practices, through GP fundholding and locality commissioning, to primary care groups, and now with the prospect of yet different organisational structures on the horizon, the role of the general practitioner has extended to include: the provision of a wider range of services requiring different clinical skills; teamworking with an increasing variety of healthcare workers; and the commissioning and quality assurance of care. This has brought general practitioners and health service managers much closer together, with general practitioners becoming more involved in the development of local health strategies. Health service managers appear to value this involvement by clinical generalists who are in regular contact with patients, are responsible for a population (the practice list) and are used to making decisions on the basis of imprecise information.[2] With the abolition of GP fundholding and the establishment of primary care trusts, general practitioners have again had to redefine their role and establish new relationships, particularly with nursing and social service colleagues and patients, who are now taking a much greater part in commissioning.

No longer can general practitioners forecast the pattern of their working lives much beyond a few years. The driving forces behind the changes of the last few years are not abating. In particular, consumerism is alive and well; technology is developing apace; the pace of new government policies is not slackening; and the financial constraints on the NHS remain. And just as general practice, primary care and the NHS are changing, so too is the new generation of general practitioners. The majority are now women and they all 'want a life', as well as a job.

What will we need?

The simple answer is that adequate numbers of caring, competent and motivated general practitioners will be needed in every part of the country.

These general practitioners of the future must be 'lifelong learners' if they are to remain caring and competent and avoid burnout, for they will be required to adapt to changes throughout their professional lives. Many will undertake research, education and management as ways of developing themselves and keeping refreshed. In this way general practice can develop as a learning organisation,[3] part of the learning society envisaged by the Dearing Report on higher education.[4] In the process, the academic discipline that is general practice will be enhanced, with more general practitioners becoming engaged in research in particular and in the development of scholarship in general.

Yet scholarship on its own will not be enough. Leadership is also required. Some general practitioners will need to develop as leaders, even though this goes against the grain in a profession that primarily fosters relationships between peers. But the new primary care organisations, let alone the wider NHS, require the qualities inherent in leadership – clarity of purpose, drive, enthusiasm, and the ability to communicate and motivate – attributes which may best be provided by general practitioners. Witness those general practitioners who have been successful in positions of leadership within NHS organisations. They have several advantages, not least their generalist clinical experience with patients. They have no vested interest in any particular patient group, unlike their specialist colleagues. They are used to listening and explaining and to making decisions usually by consensus (with patients in the consultations). They appreciate the contributions of other professions and services and they are not disconcerted by the use of medical jargon – a disadvantage occasionally suffered by lay managers confronted by clinicians. The challenge to GP educationalists and health authorities is to develop more such leaders from among the ranks of general practitioners.

Adequate numbers

Only a few years ago, at a meeting of postgraduate deans and directors of postgraduate GP education in the summer of 1997, the following stark question was posed – will more or fewer general practitioners be needed in the future? At that time no clear answer emerged from the ensuing discussion, a debate which took place in many similar meetings across the country with often equally inconclusive results. It is only in the last two years that the looming crisis in general practitioner numbers has become so evident, such that the NHS Plan promises 2000 more general practitioners and 450 (later revised to 550) extra doctors in training for general practice by 2004.[5] And in many parts even these numbers are not believed to be enough.

The fall in recruitment to vocational training schemes over the last decade is well documented. Figures for the UK show a fall of 15% between the 1988 total of 2165 and the 1994 total of 1840. These figures conceal a 31% fall in male GP registrars and a 4% rise in female GP registrars, who in 1994 comprised the majority at 55% of the total.[6]

This fall in the numbers of doctors in training for general practice has compounded other trends, leading to real difficulties for practices in some areas wishing to replace and/or recruit general practitioners.[7] These other factors include: the apparent unreadiness of graduates of vocational training to become principals in practice, at least immediately; the increased proportion of GP principals wanting to work part time or to take career breaks, usually for family reasons; and the earlier retirement of established principals.[8]

From 1990 to 1994 the number of general practitioners entering general practice fell (from 1565 to 1400), as did the number leaving practice (from 1488 to 1115). The net effect was a tiny increase, just over 1% in both the total and full-time equivalent general practitioners (from 26 757 to 27 063 full-time equivalents).[6]

Various reasons for the apparent loss of popularity of general practice have been cited, including low morale, workload, bureaucracy and out-of-hours on-call work.[8] To these might be added: increased demand from a better-informed public; the rise of consumerism and a complaints culture; the emergence of 'evidence-based medicine'; the need for greater transparency and accountability in matters of quality of care; the threat of substitution by nurses or other paramedical staff; the increased influence of health services management; and the negative impact of the popular GP press.

In their workforce plans, health authorities (at least in the Northern region) have been working on the following, admittedly crude, assumptions: that on average general practitioners will retire at age 60; that the increase in part-time working will continue; and that the total number of whole-time equivalents will rise slowly. Health authorities do not foresee a significant impact for nurse substitution, nor a need for a significant increase in whole-time equivalent general practitioners. However, they do predict, with the increased part-time working, that as many as 1.5 new general practitioners will be required to replace each retiring whole-time equivalent. The assumed increase in part-time working in general practice covers both general practitioners who spend more time with their families or in leisure pursuits and those who undertake other activities in the NHS.[8] Adequate numbers, therefore, depend on a steady increase in the recruitment of general practitioners.

There are constraints on this, which are being recognised, but which need to be addressed, particularly the number and distribution of training placements – firstly training practices. There may be sufficient training capacity in general practice nationally to meet the target increases in GP registrars for the first two years (150 in the first year and a further 200 in the second year), but not enough thereafter (for the further 200 in the following years). Furthermore, any current surplus training capacity is in the 'wrong place', i.e. in the south of England, whereas the 'under-doctored' regions are all in the north – Trent, North-West, West Midlands, and Northern and Yorkshire (Table 16.1). Between them these regions are short of 514 general practitioners (the figures relate to whole-time equivalent unrestricted principals), but only have capacity to train an additional 128. The rest of England has capacity to train an additional 236, but already has an 'excess' of 516.

Table 16.1 Distribution of GPs

Region	GPs per 100 000 weighted population	Target no. GPs for region	Distance from target – no. GPs
Northern and Yorkshire	50.5	3477	–113
Trent	49.5	2760	–144
East	53.7	2707	77
London	52.7	3762	40
South-East	55.1	4292	236
South-West	55.5	2607	163
West Midlands	51.2	2799	–54
North-West	49.3	3616	–203
England	52.2		

This inter-regional skewed distribution of need versus capacity is also visible within regions.

Secondly, the availability to the training schemes of appropriate SHO placements in hospitals is limited. The number of SHO placements directly linked to schemes, i.e. appointed by schemes, needs to be increased to allow young doctors to be appointed to programmes of training encompassing their general practice and hospital placements.

Caring, competent and motivated

We have argued that the general practitioners of the future will need to continue to learn throughout their professional lives, both to be able to cope with the changes they will encounter and to sustain their morale. They will need to be adept in five broad areas (Box 16.1).

> **Box 16.1** Skills required of GP tomorrow
>
> - Managing self.
> - Consulting with patients.
> - Working with others.
> - Maintaining good practice.
> - Relating to the public.

Managing self

In previous decades there was a greater degree of certainty and stability for general practitioners, who could reasonably anticipate their personal and professional lives, their income, their status and their place in the community. Now everyone, including general practitioners, faces change.

The cycle of stress is well described, whereby change or threat of change induces stress, which adversely affects performance, which induces more stress. To sustain their mental wellbeing and performance, general practitioners will need to be able to 'manage me first' and avoid maladaptive behaviours.

This approach demands the development of a set of attitudes, knowledge and skills such that general practitioners of the future can achieve an appropriate balance between their personal and professional lives; direct their own learning and continuing development throughout professional life; seek and find support from others when needed; be open to new ideas; reflect on their practice; and have fun as well.

General practice offers variety and even a 'portfolio career'. General practitioners can step out for at least some of their time into teaching, research or management and they can do this while holding on to their 'career anchor' of being a family doctor (*see* Chapter 15). Few others, in any field, have such opportunities.

Consulting with patients

Consulting with patients is the core activity of general practice and from this is derived its purpose and values. Despite the advances in medical science, the problems that patients bring to the privacy of the consulting room remain largely unchanged. There is an extensive literature on the consultation skills required, which include, in particular, communication and problem solving based on sound clinical reasoning. The context of clinical practice provides the ethical backdrop for general practitioners to contribute to the NHS, not least as patient advocates.

And no general practitioner, however senior, who has watched a video of themselves consulting could be fully satisfied. Enhancement of consulting skills for undergraduates, within vocational training and as part of the continuing professional development of established general practitioners, remains of continuing importance. Arguably, this applies to all doctors, not just general practitioners.

Furthermore, with the rapid expansion of information and information systems, general practitioners will need to learn how to improve the integration of information and evidence into the consultation. In the future, patients will have equal access through the Internet to medical databases. The computer terminal in the consulting room will increasingly become the third party in what Ian Purves has called the 'triadic' consultation (*see* Chapter 3), where the patient is the storyteller, the computer provides the evidence and the doctor endeavours to understand and interpret both.

Working with others

Good patient care depends on collaboration, not only between individual practitioners but also between organisations. Thus, general practitioners need to be able to work effectively with other doctors, nurses, counsellors, physiotherapists, practices, primary care trusts, health authorities, hospitals and social service departments. Teamworking is essential, but critically dependent on valuing colleagues and understanding their roles.[9]

Good teams also require leadership and good management. It will fall to general practitioners to provide this in many instances. Leadership is not a divine right and needs to be earned. Seniority is not a satisfactory criterion; the senior partner is not necessarily the most able leader.

Maintaining good practice

As professionals, general practitioners are responsible for maintaining their own professional standards. Through revalidation this will need be done transparently to be able to achieve the levels of accountability expected by government, public and professional colleagues alike.

As Sir Donald Irvine has noted,[10] general practitioners are most able to maintain good practice when they work in teams which: show leadership; have clear values and standards; are collectively committed to sustaining and improving quality; foster learning; have a 'no blame' culture; and are prepared for external review. Such teams use a range of effective management practices to assure quality, including clinical guidelines and protocols, having good record and information systems, education and training, systematic clinical audit, and appraisal and mentoring.

Here evidence can be harnessed for the care of patients, and the quality of the care provided for specific groups, for example patients with diabetes, can be demonstrated. This process can be further enhanced by the use of appropriate information technology, particularly where it supports care of individuals by multidisciplinary clinical teams.

Relating to the public

Primary care, including general practice, is a public service responding very largely to public demand. In an age of consumerism and government plan, general practitioners and their colleagues in primary care are adjusting to new demands for responsiveness, accessibility and service. And there is much to learn from the techniques employed by commercial service industries and from patients.

Yet the commercial analogy cannot be pushed too far. Being a customer is different from being a patient and the relationship between doctor and patient is governed by a different set of customs and rules. These customs and rules have, however, changed over the last few years and the 'bargain' between general practitioner and patient is no longer as clear as it was. There is, however, very real substance in the doctor–patient relationship, but the relationship does need both to enable and accommodate dynamic change.[11]

General practitioners will need particular skills to negotiate and renegotiate the 'bargain' with patients, both with individuals and with the public at large. They will also need to ensure that they and their colleagues employ the best anti-discriminatory practices, to avoid creating disadvantage in healthcare on the basis of gender, race, sexuality or disability.

What needs to be done?

In summary, then, the general practitioners of the future will need to be generalists, clinicians, team players, lifelong learners and managers (at least of themselves). Some will need to provide leadership. The difficulties in recruitment, the apparent unreadiness of GP registrars to become principals on completion of vocational training, the presence of poor morale and the consequent impaired performance among existing general practitioners mean that action is required to revitalise general practice as a career for the twenty-first century.

Before full registration

There has been much debate on the selection of medical students. Is an ability to gain high marks in A-level sciences an appropriate entry criterion for a profession that is both science- and humanity-based? General practice, in particular, might believe that this bias towards science would prejudice students against pursuing a career in such a 'humane' speciality. It appears, however, that experiences during, rather than before, medical education are the more critical determinants of ultimate career choice.

Indeed, an attachment of at least six weeks full time in general practice late in the undergraduate years, particularly if the experience is a good one, seems an important influence in choosing general practice as a career.[12] The widespread increase in community-based teaching, primarily in general practice, in the curricula of most medical schools, particularly the new medical schools, should be beneficial to general practitioner recruitment in the future. General practitioners engaged in this teaching must ensure that the experience is a positive one. Poor teaching and exposure to cynicism or negativity drive students away.

Equally, the relatively new development of pre-registration house officer posts in general practice should benefit not only those who ultimately become general practitioners, but also those who become specialists. With the rapid increase of day case procedures, many surgical posts now offer only limited opportunities for young doctors to learn the duties of a doctor[13] and general practice is arguably a more appropriate clinical setting. The logistical problems of providing all pre-registration doctors with a period in general practice are immense and are unlikely to be overcome in the next five years. The 'modernisation' of the SHO grade, however, offers the promise that general practice might become an integral component of the generic first year of all doctors' foundation programmes.

Vocational training

Although vocational training for general practice is considered a success story, it appears that a proportion of doctors completing it are unready for life as a principal. The establishment of national summative assessment does assure minimum clinical competence for independent practice, but there is clearly more to being a general practitioner. The three years' duration of vocational training was always a compromise, particularly as only one year is spent in general practice.[14] It remains to be seen whether an extended period in practice would equip doctors better for becoming a principal immediately, though the case has been well argued.[15] The extra six months would need to concentrate not only on the further development of consultation skills, but also on other necessary skills (Box 16.1) if the gap between registrar and principal is to be bridged.

Induction and higher professional education

Rather than extend the period of vocational training, the Royal College of General Practitioners and others have argued that it should be augmented by a period of 'higher professional education'.[15] This was first proposed by the College in 1985, though the length of the period was not prescribed.[14] The College stated that a minimum period of two years would seem appropriate, as recent developments in practice had exposed the limitations of the three-year vocational training period. Education in the clinical area, health service and practice organisation and management, team working, audit and quality assurance, research and teaching all demand a longer training period.

Albeit for different motivations, the various post-vocational training schemes have provided young general practitioners with an opportunity for 'higher professional education' and induction into practice. In Durham, the motivation was a recruitment crisis; in the North-West, it was the raising of standards and recruitment. In Lambeth, Southwark and Lewisham, the motivation was also recruitment, whereas for the London Academic Training Scheme, it was the development of general practice as an academic discipline.

Whatever the primary reason, each scheme appears to be meeting a need in young doctors and providing some stimulus to local practitioners and practices to develop, as well as recruiting young doctors to work in deprived areas, with some pursuing an academic career.

There are features common to all the schemes which deserve to be heeded (Box 16.2). First, the young doctors involved become 'fit for purpose' (that is, able to work as a principal) as opposed to 'fit for practice' (that is, independent clinical practice following vocational training and certified through summative assessment) or 'fit for award' (as for a higher qualification). Second, the schemes offer personal and collective support for personal development through mentoring and small group learning. And third, the schemes provide a flexible and supportive induction to the real world of general practice (as opposed to the refined world of training practices!).

Box 16.2 Common features of post-vocational training schemes

- Develop fitness for purpose.
- Use mentoring and group learning.
- Provide induction to the real world.

A period of higher professional education for general practitioners should be an induction to becoming a principal (or their future equivalent), a transition from being a registrar.[15] The period need not be prescribed, as it is designed to equip individual doctors to be 'fit for purpose'. In these circumstances, there is no single form of certification of completion that would be appropriate, though arguably Membership of the Royal College of General Practitioners (MRCGP) could be so developed for the majority in the future.

Continuing professional development

The generic skills required of general practitioners in the future (Box 16.1) will need constant refreshment. Indeed, these skills presuppose a different approach to continued learning based on reflection and self-directed towards need. Yet the present diet of continuing medical education (CME) for many general practitioners is still based on accreditation of courses for Postgraduate Education Allowance (PGEA). It pays little heed to either the assessment of doctors' educational needs or the effective evaluation of outcome and its impact on performance.[16] Programmes are heavily dominated by pharmaceutical companies, who provide sponsorship, and inevitably concentrate on disease management and drug therapy. Patients and health service managers have little or no say in what is essentially a 'professionals-only' activity.

This is changing, and it needs to.[17] In future, programmes must better reflect the needs of practitioners, patients and the health service, and sustain the broader notion of continuing professional development. No longer can they concentrate narrowly on CME, and be private occupational therapy for doctors. Continuing professional development will help doctors as they contend with the demands of patient expectations, changing clinical practice and new organisational structures. Other forms of learning incorporated in personal development plans should progressively replace the lecture format, which was so favoured in the past.[18] Regular appraisal and revalidation, mid-career breaks, sabbaticals and involvement in other professional activities (teaching, research and management) will all contribute, and increasing numbers of general practitioners may be expected to undertake a wider range of higher qualifications, from certificate to doctoral level – a trend which is visible now but was largely absent in the past.

And some doctors, presumed to be a tiny minority, will require remedial training because their performance has fallen below acceptable minimum standards. These doctors may be identified either by their peers as primary care trusts start to grapple with the issue of clinical governance. The trusts may be expected to concentrate on those doctors whose quality of care is poor and whose use of resources is wasteful, and they may be well placed to use incentives from more efficient use of resources to support these colleagues (and their patients). In this way management of the service, quality of patient care and professional education might become better aligned. The National Clinical Assessment Authority and the Directors of Postgraduate GP Education will need to help by providing expertise in assessment and remediation.

Future themes for GPs tomorrow

For general practice, all of this suggests a number of strategic themes for the coming decade – leadership, scholarship and fellowship (Box 16.3). Each of these requires new and flexible approaches for its development.

Box 16.3 Strategic themes for GPs tomorrow

Leadership
- vision
- communication skill
- motivating others
- above vested interests.

Scholarship
- learning valued
- research and teaching
- higher qualifications.

Fellowship
- mutual support
- flexible careers
- mentoring.

Leadership

For many general practitioners the recent period of change has resulted in more work, more pressure and more uncertainty.[19] Many have relished this, but some have felt ill-equipped to survive, let alone thrive. The challenge for the future is finding ways to enable general practitioners not only to manage change, but to lead it. This requires the ability to shape, share and articulate vision and strategy, excellent communication skills, drive and enthusiasm, political awareness, and the ability to motivate and support others. These GP leaders must rise above parochial and professional vested interests. Leadership is neither wholly an innate quality nor wholly a learned skill. Some doctors have an aptitude to become leaders and they need opportunities to develop the appropriate skills.[20]

Scholarship

General practice is an academic discipline with a body of professional knowledge it can legitimately call its own. In the past, some service general practitioners have inclined to be dismissive of their academic colleagues, but this is changing. More now recognise that they learn throughout their professional life and have come to value learning as a means of personal growth and professional development.

The enhanced opportunities for becoming involved in teaching, particularly medical student teaching, and research and the wider range of higher qualifications available means that general practice in the future will have a much stronger cadre of academically experienced doctors. This will help provide the discipline with the necessary resources to handle change and, more importantly, the necessary knowledge and skills to develop more effective patient care.

Fellowship

There is no politically correct equivalent word and, in this context, fellowship does not refer to Fellowship (of the Royal College of General Practitioners) by Assessment. It is that environment of collegiality and mutual support that should characterise general practice and primary care in the future, an environment where each individual values the other for their contribution and where different kinds of personal support are available. In such an environment, flexible training and work patterns will be encouraged; collective learning and co-counselling (and similar techniques) will be widely used; mentoring and appraisal will be commonplace; and portfolio careers and different employment options will be expected. Stress will be acknowledged and dealt with, not hidden or denied. A range of means will be used to overcome professional isolation, not only of doctors in the remote rural areas but also of those stranded alone in the inner city.

Cynics may say that the NHS will never provide the necessary resources or protected time to support this more structured approach to professional development. But much has already been achieved through partnership between general practice and health authorities. And much more may yet be gained from the opportunities which arise from the 'new NHS'.

Summary

- General practice will continue to have a critical role in the NHS.
- General practitioners will need to be adept at managing themselves, consulting with patients and working with others.
- Action is required on a number of fronts to ensure adequate numbers of caring, competent and motivated general practitioners.
- The development of leadership, scholarship and fellowship is needed to sustain general practice in the future.

References

1 Department of Health (2001) *Shifting the Balance of Power within the NHS: securing delivery.* Cnmd 3807. Department of Health, London.
2 Smith J and Shapiro J (1997) *Holding on While Letting Go.* Health Services Management Centre, Birmingham.
3 Marquardt M and Reynolds A (1994) *The Global Learning Organisation.* Irwin, New York.
4 National Committee of Inquiry into Higher Education (1997) *Higher Education in the Learning Society.* HMSO, London.
5 Secretary of State for Health (2000) *The NHS Plan: a plan for investment, a plan for reform.* The Stationery Office, London.
6 Taylor DH and Leese B (1997) Recruitment, retention, and time commitment change of general practitioners in England and Wales, 1990–4: a retrospective study. *BMJ.* **314**: 1806–10.
7 Medical Practices Committee (1995) *General Practice Recruitment Survey.* MPC, London.
8 Royal College of General Practitioners (1997) *The Primary Care Workforce – a descriptive analysis.* RCGP, London.
9 Pearson P and Spencer J (eds) (1997) *Promoting Teamwork in Primary Care. A Research Based Approach.* Arnold, London.
10 Irvine D (1997) Maintaining good practice: protecting patients from poor performance. *BMJ.* **314**: 1613–15.

11   van Zwanenberg T (2001) The new GP. In: J Harrison, R Innes and T van Zwanenberg (eds) *The New GP: changing roles and the modern NHS*. Radcliffe Medical Press, Oxford.

12   Sullivan FM and Morrison JM (1997) What can universities do to reverse the decline in the numbers of doctors entering general practice? *Medical Education.* **31**: 235–6.

13   General Medical Council (1995) *Duties of a Doctor*. GMC, London.

14   Royal College of General Practitioners (1994) *Education and Training for General Practice*. RCGP, London.

15   van Zwanenberg T, Pringle M, Smail S, Baker M and Field S (2001) The case for strengthening education and training for general practice. *British Journal of General Practice.* **51**: 349–50.

16   Department of Health (1998) *A Review of Continuing Professional Development in General Practice*. Department of Health, London.

17   Richards T (1998) Continuing medical education. Needs to be more effective, accountable and responsive to all stakeholders in health. *BMJ.* **316**: 246.

18   Sylvester S (2001) Continuing professional development. In: J Harrison, R Innes and T van Zwanenberg (eds) *The New GP: changing roles and the modern NHS*. Radcliffe Medical Press, Oxford.

19   Irvine D (1993) General practice in the 1990s: a personal view on future developments. *British Journal of General Practice.* **43**: 121–5.

20   Harrison J (2000) Developing leaders. In: T van Zwanenberg and J Harrison (eds) *Clinical Governance in Primary Care*. Radcliffe Medical Press, Oxford.

CHAPTER 17

Conclusion – new flexibilities

Jamie Harrison

You can never plan the future by the past.
Edmund Burke

This concluding chapter summarises the key messages of the book. Although life may be uncertain, the GPs of tomorrow will develop flexible careers, with confidence in their own abilities and in what they have to offer patients and the wider world of medicine.

1948 versus 1998 and beyond

Much has changed in the 50 years since the inception of the NHS. The initial scepticism and suspicion of doctors about the NHS have given way to an increasing ownership of its values and priorities, not least in providing personal and continuing medical care, free at the point of contact, to patients.

Yet, perhaps as never before, question marks surround the future funding of the service, the scope of treatments it will be able to offer and the working patterns and morale of its staff, not least its doctors. Will they increasingly become technicians with communication skills or will the one-to-one doctor–patient relationship, with its pastoral care, remain the corner-stone, as patients desire (Chapter 14)?

Experience from the various post-vocational training schemes (Chapters 7–9) suggests that general practice is safe in the hands of young doctors, who are keen to develop personally and professionally. Moreover, they have begun to challenge the status quo where it has failed to provide proper models of career development.

Old wisdom

It is all too easy to be critical of younger doctors who no longer wish to practise in the traditional way. Long hours on call, the continuous demand of patients and the apparent inflexibility of a medical partnership deter many from a conventional GP career. Yet these doctors are just as committed to medicine, as Chapter 13 demonstrates.

Previous generations of general practitioners have valued their contractual arrangements, which stemmed from the 1948 settlement. Partnership has given them stability, fellowship and the freedom to choose partners and implement decisions.

These 'old flexibilities' will remain attractive to some, though the responsibility and freedom they provide will seem overwhelming to others. A transition to innovative types of partnership, which might employ a number of doctors and where becoming a partner only comes with time and an expressed desire, may bridge the gap between old and new.

New flexibilities

The focus of much of the book has been on the perceived need of younger general practitioners to discover a fulfilling way to pursue a life in general practice. This has involved finding stepping stones (Chapters 7 and 8) into practice life. Such induction into general practice has involved developing new skills and learning about research (Chapter 9) or grappling with new sorts of salaried post (Chapter 10).

Older practitioners have also responded to the chance to renew their enthusiasm for general practice with mid-career support (Chapter 11) and through the experience of being mentors. Exposure to the younger generation has stimulated questions about how to be a general practitioner in the twenty-first century.

New flexibilities include working arrangements which provide protected time for study, support, recreation and family life. New primary care organisations are emerging as employers of general practitioners; they may have their drawbacks. A loss of autonomy and limited freedom to make local decisions quickly and effectively may result. Equally, these organisations will not run with slack in the system. Difficult decisions about taking sick and maternity leave will continue. And patient expectations will remain.

What is flexible working for one person may be slavery for another. Regaining control of their career (Chapter 15) should allow individual doctors the freedom to map out their own destinies, while adhering to the ethos and values of traditional general practice.

New partnerships

Much debate will continue on whether medical partnership as the model for general practice is now outdated. New networks are emerging which may provide new ways of bringing general practitioners together. What is clear, however, is that other sorts of partnership are also beginning to form.

Primary care organisations (PCOs) and general practitioners will increasingly work together, through 'career start' type schemes (Chapter 7) and other salaried options (Chapter 10) – a trend set to accelerate with the development of PCTs (Chapter 2). Alliances between medical educationalists, local medical committees and health authorities signal one way forward in developing the GP career of tomorrow, founded on the triad of leadership, scholarship and fellowship (Chapter 16). For general practitioners can no longer exist in isolation, from their peers, their patients, their colleagues or from mechanisms to enhance their own personal growth.

Increasingly, partnerships with other healthcare professionals, both in primary and secondary care, point the way to a seamless model of service provision. Training, learning and planning together should encourage greater trust and confidence with which to face the difficult decisions affecting the health service of the future.

Last, but very much not least, come partnerships with patients. Young doctors continue to value their role in patient care (Chapter 13) but rightly question some of the paternalism and medicalisation of the past (Chapter 1). These doctors have the opportunity to consult with intelligence and effectiveness, harnessing the power of information technology and smarter ways of working (Chapter 3). For consultation with patients will remain at the heart of general practice, however, the style and context of such consultations may be modified by teamworking and delegation.

Conclusion

The *Shorter Oxford English Dictionary* defines the word 'doctor' (initially in its archaic use) as 'a teacher, instructor; one who inculcates learning, opinions or principles'. The dictionary goes on to state this usage is now rare. Yet this early expression of what it means to be a doctor has continuing relevance for general practitioners.

The good teacher will remain eager to keep on learning and conscious of the need to maintain a balanced life, both intellectually and personally. For only when the individual doctor is healthy can 'learning, opinions and principles' be properly passed on to others.

The general practitioners of tomorrow will face continuing pressures to meet targets and deadlines and the needs of ill people. Portions of their time will be demanded by managers, patients and their own families. But hopefully they will also be the wise ones, who have learned to make time for their own needs – for recreation, reflection and participation in all that it means to be truly human.

Index